613.7

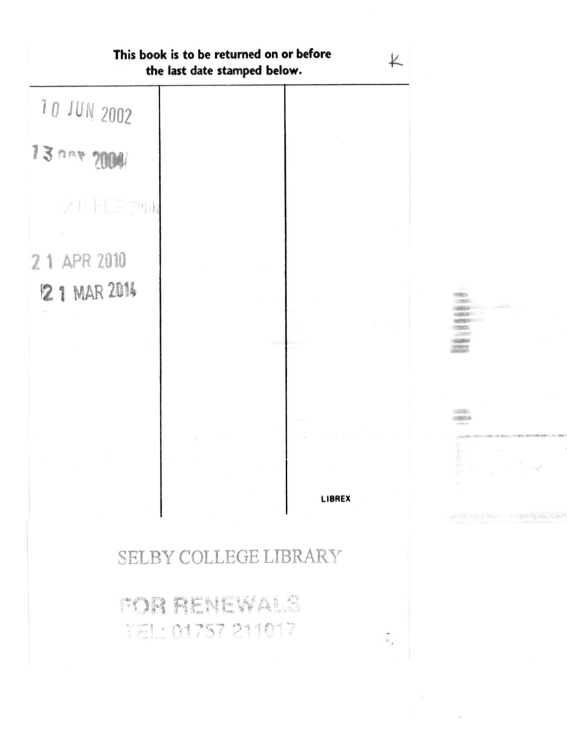

the beginner's guide to
Tai Chi

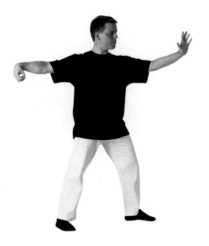

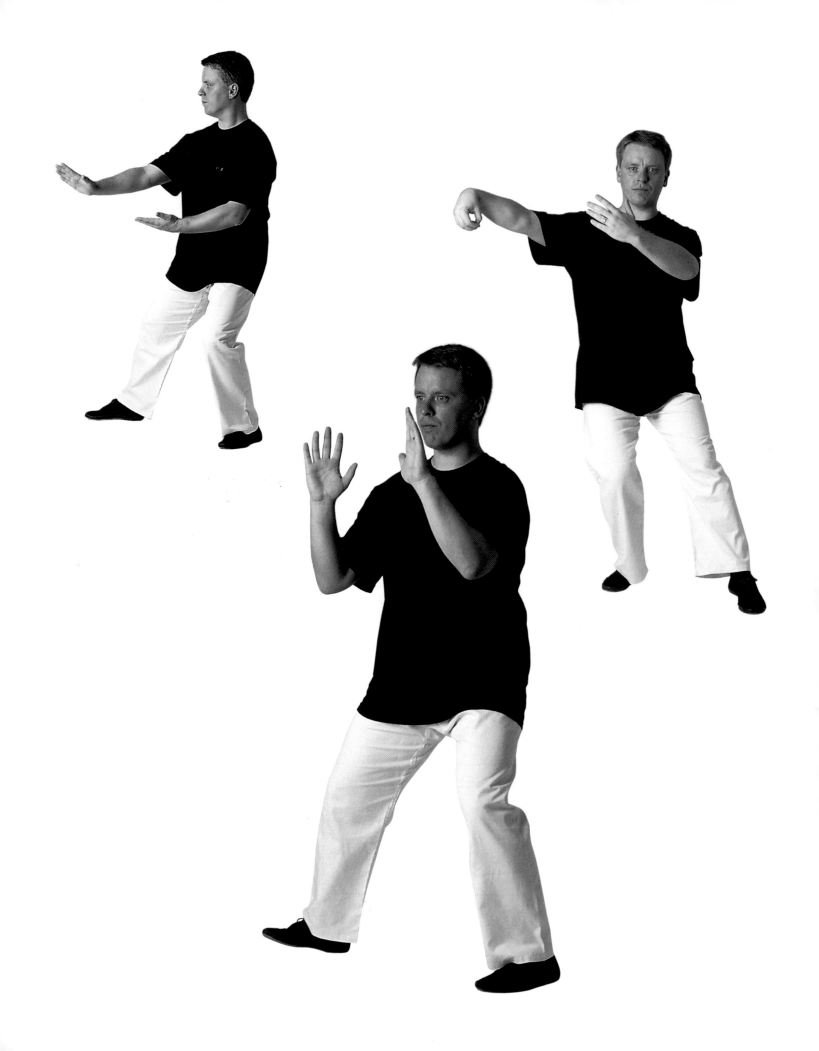

the beginner's guide to
Tai Chi

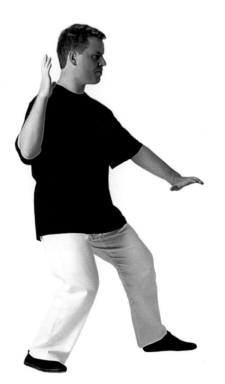

Ray Pawlett

D&S

BOOKS

First published in 2001 by D&S Books

© 2001 D&S Books

D&S Books
Cottage Meadow, Bocombe,
Parkham, Bideford
Devon, England
EX39 5PH

e-mail us at:- enquiries.dspublishing@care4free.net

This edition printed 2001

ISBN 1-903327-16-4
Editorial Director: Sarah King
Editor: Sarah Harris
Project Editor: Judith Millidge
Photographer: Paul Forrester
Designer: Axis Design Editions Limited

Distributed in the UK & Ireland by
Bookmart Limited
Desford Road
Enderby
Leicester LE9 5AD

Distributed in Australia by
Herron Books
39 Commercial Road
Fortitude Valley
Queensland 4006

1 3 5 7 9 10 8 6 4 2

CONTENTS

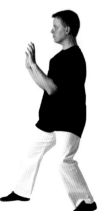

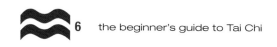
INTRODUCTION

During my years of teaching Tai Chi, I have frequently been asked if there is a good book on the subject. My answer has always been somewhat reserved. Although there are many excellent Tai Chi books available, they usually seem to comprise of little more that the form itself or a discussion of items that you will only be interested in if you have already learned the basics.

This book demonstrates section one of the traditional Yang long form, and shows you how to put more depth into your practice.

I firmly believe that it is far better to be able to do section one to a good level than it is to practice the whole form ineffectively. It will give you a sense of having achieved something real and should set up a platform for further study.

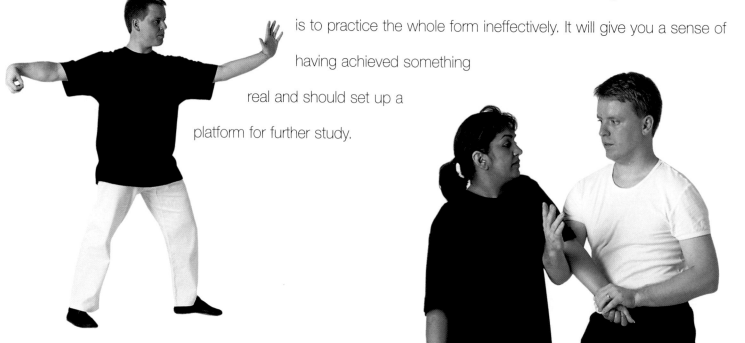

Single Whip, from the Yang style form. Learning one section of the form in depth will lead to greater undrstanding.

Although Tai Chi is not purely a 'fighting' form of martial art, you must understand martial applications.

What are martial arts?

What do you think of if you try to define the phrase 'martial arts'? If you are attracted to the idea of studying Tai Chi, then you probably do not find that the concept of martial arts as pure fighting skills provides the whole picture.

There are many arguments and discussions about what forms the essence of a martial art. I recently saw an interview with a very skilled martial artist who regarded the meditation aspects of martial arts training as pure nonsense and preferred to teach his students very dangerous techniques.

To my mind, this is not the true essence of martial arts. From my personal experience and discussion with other martial artists, most students do not simply want to learn how to fight. Healing and inner development also seem to be an underlying theme to the martial artist.

If you examine the history of martial arts, there is normally a connection with some sort of inner development that seeks higher things. For example, Tai Chi is connected to Taoism, karate and other styles, and to Buddhism. Even in English folklore the warrior Knights of the Round Table were on a spiritual quest for the Holy Grail.

An easy reply for the martial artist mentioned earlier would be, 'What good will it all do if somebody attacks you?' The truth is that if you are taken by surprise, no amount of martial training can help you. The real trick is to avoid being taken by surprise.

Most students of martial arts wish to learn more than simply fighting skills. Many have an interest in healing skills also, such as Shiatsu, shown here.

Tai Chi has connection with many other forms of martial art, including karate.

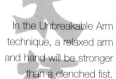

Hard and soft styles

In the world of martial arts, there is a division between two different ways of working. These are generally termed hard and soft styles. Tai Chi is known as a soft style. Remember your Taoist theory: the two styles,

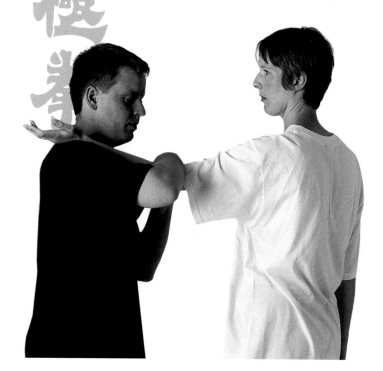

hard and soft, are a Yin and Yang pair. This means that within every hard style there is an element of softness and within every soft style there is an element of hardness. If you want an example, watch a Chen style expert. The form will comprise soft Yin movements and some very explosive Yang movements.

There is Yin and Yang within every movement that you practice. If you ever hear a martial artist claiming that hard is better than soft or vice versa, you will understand that they cannot know what they are talking about. How can one be better than the other if they all have elements of the same thing? It is far better to respect all styles. I have learned lessons that I can apply to Tai Chi from studying hard styles. So can you if you approach with an open mind.

If you can apply this to all that you do in the form, you are probably already a master!

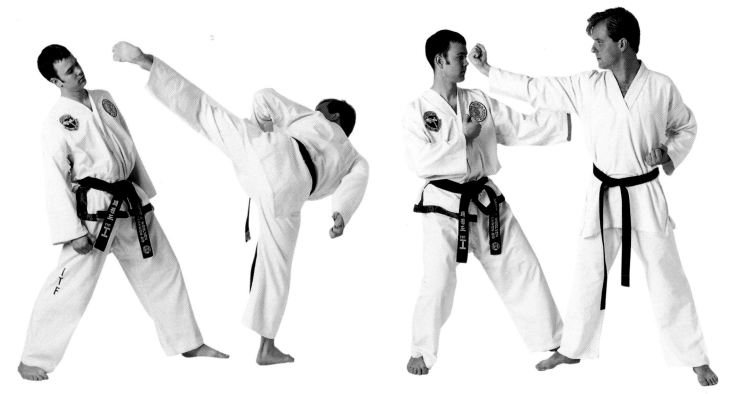

Tae Kwon Do is a well-known example of a 'hard' style of martial art. It uses many fast kicks and punches.

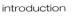

There is a general difference between hard and soft styles. In soft styles, all movement will be curved in some way. In hard styles, this need not be so. A punch will normally be straight with little or no curved path. If you imagine that hard styles are similar to pistons and rods working in straight lines and that a soft style is more like a whiplash, you will have some idea of the difference. Do not forget that there is always hard within soft, so this will not always be the perfect image, but it does give some idea.

The following exercise can help you get some idea of how soft styles work:

This experiment is merely an illustration of how softness can redirect strength. The hard style masters are also aware of this. The inner forearm block described below would be accompanied by a twisting movement in a genuine hard block, but would have the same effect.

In a 'soft' style of martial art, such as Tai Chi, softness can overcome strength. Here the yielding to a partner's punch has allowed the other opponent to gain control.

1. Stand opposite your partner who has extended their fist.

2. Press your inner forearm against their forearm as though you were blocking.

3.Y our partner should hold their arm rigid. You will feel that you need to put pressure on them to change the course of the punch and block it.

4. Now take your two front fingers and place them against your partners fist.

5. Flick the punch to one side. This should take very little effort on your part, no matter how rigidly they hold their arm.

WHAT IS TAI CHI?

Do you know what Tai Chi is? One of the amusing things about Tai Chi is that it is fairly difficult to define, yet you will find many who will delight in telling you what Tai Chi really is. I have been studying the art for several years and still find an absolute definition elusive, yet I have met many who have merely read a magazine article and are able to pinpoint a definition straight away!

The Chinese character for Tai Chi.

This is actually one of the aspects of Tai Chi. When you start learning it the definition seems fairly concrete. Yet after a few year's study when you are starting to understand better, it becomes easier to say what Tai Chi is not. One reason for this is that a detailed study of Tai Chi will affect you on so many different levels that trying to define the nature of it in words seems crude and inefficient.

Tai Chi has three sources of knowledge.

These are:

1. Martial arts
2. Healing
3. Philosophy

The history of Tai Chi shows you that the martial art side of Tai Chi is probably the vehicle that carried it to so many people. Yet if you look at the traditional masters, they all had a good knowledge of Taoism and traditional Chinese healing arts.

The connection between these seemingly diverse areas is Chi. Chi is the life force that exists within us all. If your Chi is strong, you can use it both for self-defence and healing. It will also raise the level of that part of your consciousness that lends itself to spiritual thinking and philosophy.

So I suppose if you really want a concrete definition of what Tai Chi is about, then it is a series of methods to enhance one's Chi.

This diagram clearly illustrates the three sources of knowledge, and shows how they interconnect.

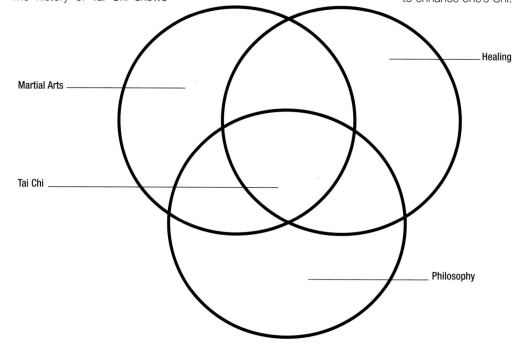

Martial Arts

Healing

Tai Chi

Philosophy

The historical background of Tai Chi

Learning the history of Tai Chi may not seem very appealing to everybody who starts to learn the art. If, however, you stop to consider the implications of Tai Chi history, then you will find it a fascinating subject. Consider, for example, that at the same time as Galileo was raising his telescope to the heavens, the patriarch of Tai Chi, Chen Wanting, was working on what would become the Tai Chi forms. And at the time when Archimedes was taking his famous bath, the concept of Yin and Yang was being defined.

The first usage of the words Tai Chi was in the *Book of Changes* dating from the Zhou Dynasty (221 BC). Tai Chi in this sense refers to the two opposites that are frequently referred to as Yin and Yang. The ideas of Yin and Yang will be explained shortly.

Chen Wanting lived in the 16th century. He served as a royal guard in his home village and was taught by a famous general in the imperial army. After the fall of the Ming Dynasty, Chen Wanting withdrew from society to further his Taoist studies. He wrote many manuscripts and taught his art to other people.

The 19th century saw the rise of Yang Luchan (1799-1872). He was born to a poor family and left home as a child to become a servant for the Chen family. Yang Luchan would watch and learn from the martial arts instructors around him. After very hard training he became a skilled martial artist.

Yang then returned to his home to lodge at a pharmacy and make a living by teaching Tai Chi. He adapted the style he had learned to make it more accessible to everyday people. The Yang style of Tai Chi was thus born. The style was later adapted both by his son, Yang Jianhou, and his grandson, Yang Chengfu. The Yang Chengfu form is that practised by the modern school of Yang practitioners.

Another of Yang Luchan's sons, Yang Banhou, invented the Wu style. This style of Tai Chi uses a slightly different way of moving but is similar in its method.

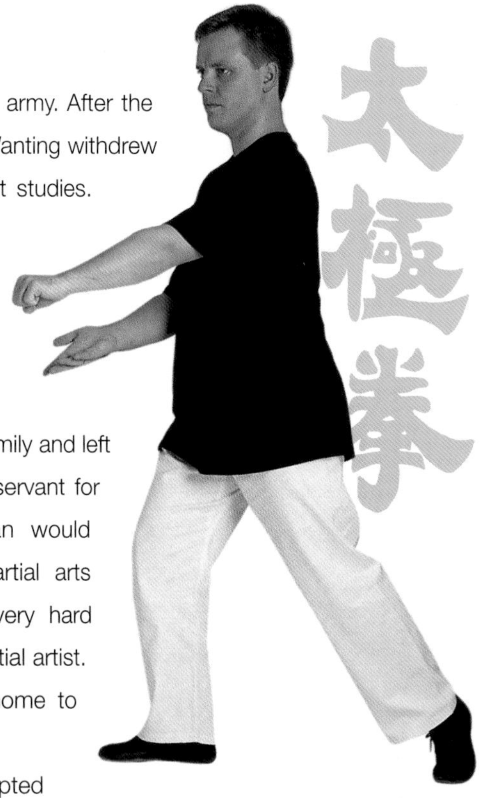

Parry, Block and Punch is a traditional move from the original Yang style of Tai Chi.

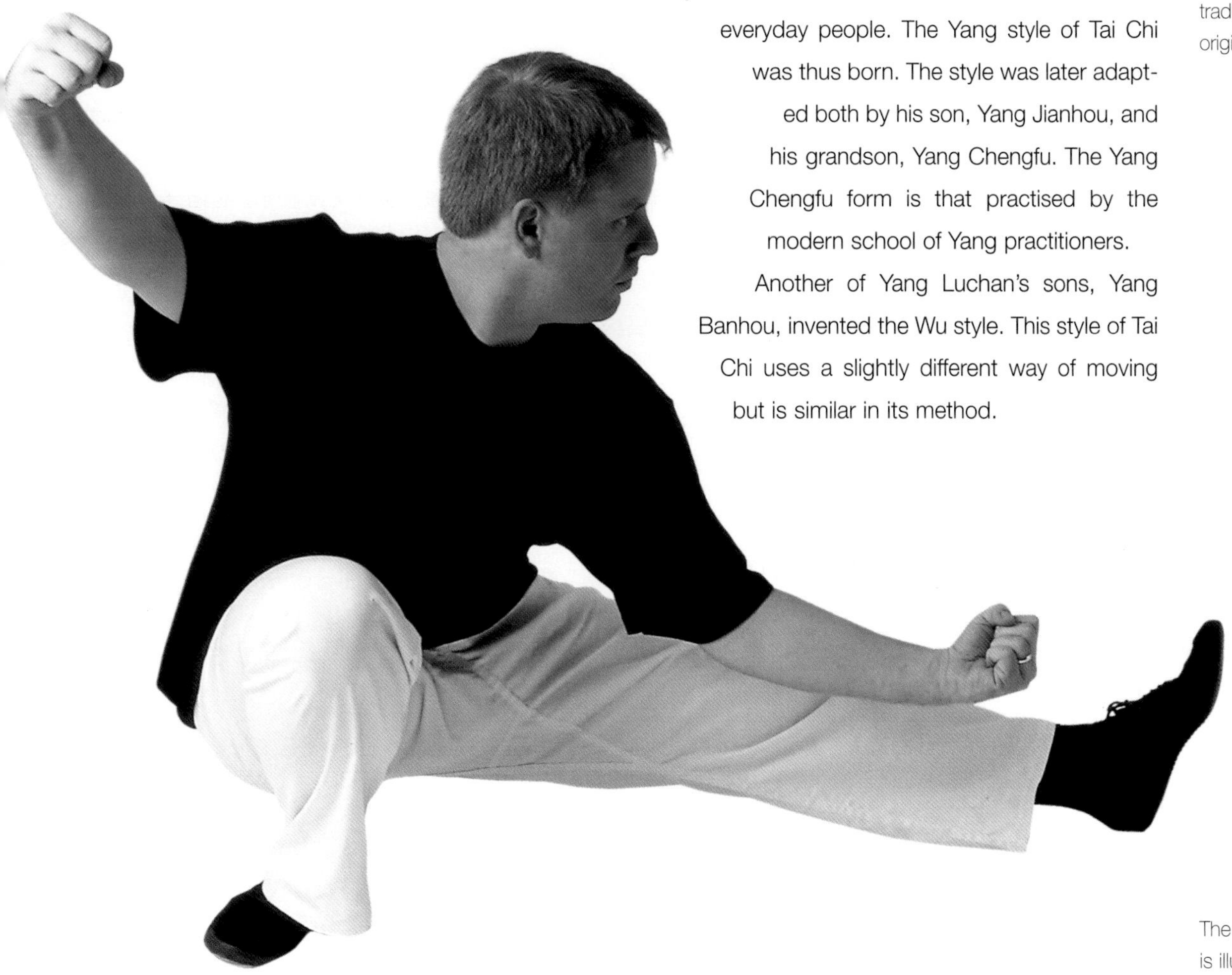

The Chen style of Tai Chi uses more explosive movements. The Dragon on the Ground is illustrated here.

The philosophical background of Tai Chi

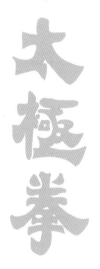

The philosophical background of Tai Chi is based on Taoism. The first thing to understand about Taoism is that it is not a religion in the sense that you are expected to worship a deity. Taoist ideas need not be at odds with any other beliefs that you may have. I know practising Christians who are very interested in Taoism and find no conflict.

Taoism stems from a desire to understand the nature of the world around us. Using tools such as meditation, the Taoists have invented concepts that describe both the universe as a whole, and man's relationship to it. Many of the revelations of the ancient Taoists are being rediscovered by modern scientists.

A central concept of Taoism is Wu Wei. Literally it means, 'without causing or making'. This definition has been somewhat altered by several thinkers. Many interpret this as meaning doing nothing. How can anything be of use if all it means is do nothing?

What it is actually means is, 'without meddlesome, combative or egotistical effort'. Think how much easier your life would be if more people managed to take this idea into their thought processes.

It is also a useful reference in Tai Chi. When you are practising Tai Chi, you only do what needs to be done. If you start adding your own embellishments, then you are not following Wu Wei. Also, if you find that your mind is wandering during the form, try thinking about the concept of Wu Wei.

When you see somebody who is skilled in an action, they make the job look easy. Yet when they ask you if you want to try, it may seem very difficult. This sort of trained attention to detail without seeming to make any effort is another manifestation of Wu Wei.

When the Taoists tried to describe their world, they looked at what nature was doing around them. They examined the ebb and flow of the seasons and how they affected our lives on various levels. From this, they constructed a model of the world that is known as 'Five Element theory'.

Five Element theory is just one of many models for describing the world. If you have others that you prefer it does not matter. The concept behind the theory is that the world consists of the five elements, fire, earth, metal, water and wood.

They all react with one another in a myriad of different ways. Each element will also have a set of body organs attributed to it. Their mutual interaction is also described in Five Element theory.

A major part of Taoist theory is the idea of Yin and Yang. The well-known black and white symbol that most call the Yin Yang symbol is actually called the Tai Chi symbol. The concept of Yin and Yang is so entwined within Tai Chi theory that it is worth taking a slightly deeper look at it.

Diagram showing the relationships between the Five Elements.

Yin and Yang

Yin and Yang are the cornerstones of Taoist philosophy and Tai Chi theory. They are the two polarities that emerged from the 'original Chi'.

Yin is expressed as contracting, passive, cold, water, dark, receptive, the Moon, female, emotions, etc. Yin is usually contraction and flowing downwards. It is the composition of intelligence.

Yang is expansive, active, hot, fire, light, giving, the Sun, male, creativity, etc. Yang is expansive and rising. It is the expression of intelligence.

Within Yin, there is Yang and within Yang, there is Yin. There is no absolute Yin or Yang; they are relative to one another. They will always change at the extremes, e.g. Yin will become Yang and Yang will become Yin.

In the Tai Chi form, there is always expansion and contraction. These are the forces of Yin and Yang being expressed within the form. Remember that you cannot have Yin without Yang. Therefore if you have rising energy, such as in the White Crane movement, you will also need sinking energy in the legs.

White Crane Spreads its Wings is a good example of Yin and Yang within Tai Chi. You have both rising energy in the arms, and sinking energy in the legs.

The famous Yin and Yang symbol.

Tai Chi as a martial art

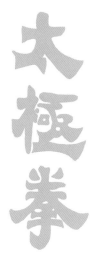

Tai Chi is a complete martial arts system. It contains blocks, strikes, locks, escapes and vital point knowledge. It is all hidden away in the form for those who understand it. This is why even a simple looking movement can have many applications.

The style of Tai Chi that you practice should make little difference to your long-term goals. People with different body requirements invented the different styles. For example the Chen style has lower postures than the Yang style and is therefore more demanding on your legs. The long-term goals however remain constant.

In Tai Chi it is always assumed that if you need to defend yourself, it will be against a bigger and stronger aggressor. The techniques therefore use softness rather than strength. Some believe that the inherent soft or Yin qualities make the art particularly suitable for women. There have been many women who have reached very high skill levels in Tai Chi.

Tee shirt and shorts or jogging pants are ideal for practicing Tai Chi. Simple plimsolls make the best footwear, although you can practise barefoot.

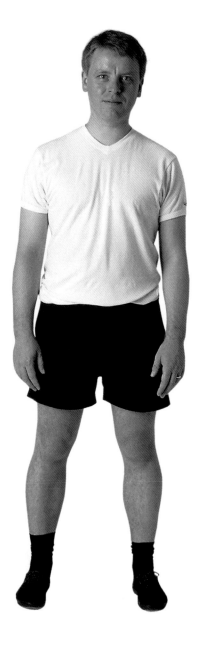

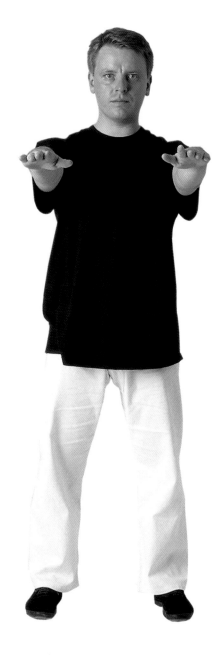

If you practise Tai Chi, you are unlikely to gain any injuries from your lesson. In some styles free sparring can be dangerous if not controlled. In Tai Chi, free sparring is replaced by pushing hands. Some hard styles also practice destruction techniques. This means breaking thing with different parts of your body. This is not a feature of Tai Chi, so you do not have to worry about bruised knuckles!

In Tai Chi, you do not try to fight force with force. This would result in the strongest person winning every time. Instead we use the principle of yielding. If an Energy is coming towards you, you should let it come, but neutralise or redirect it.

You do not need much to start practising Tai Chi. Most students will train in either jogging trousers or shorts and a tee shirt. There is no need for a special outfit unless you enter a Tai Chi tournament. Training shoes are not ideal for Tai Chi practice. This is because they are generally designed for running, and have built-up heels. A better and cheaper

option is to use old-fashioned plimsolls or deck shoes. 'Kung Fu slippers,' have come onto the market in recent years, but are normally overpriced. Avoid the ones that have hard plastic soles, as these can slip on hard floors.

If you study Tai Chi the martial aspect should be fun. Stay focused on what you are doing but do not be afraid to enjoy yourself. If you are happy, then your body will be more relaxed and your Tai Chi will work better.

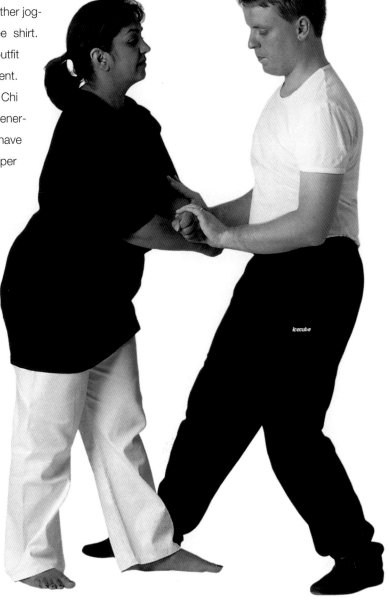

In the Press movement, from Grasping the Sparrow's Tail, yielding is used instead of force to redirect the energy from an opponent's attack.

Tai Chi as a healing art

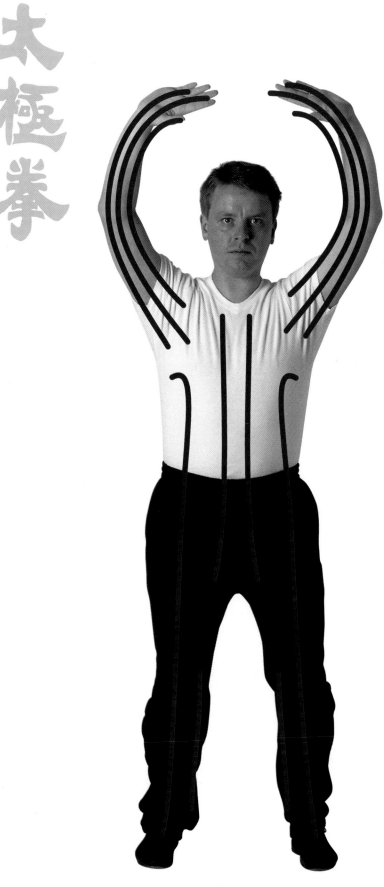

Remember how we said at the end of the last chapter that Tai Chi works better if you are relaxed? And that if you are happy, you will be more relaxed? This should already be giving some sort of indication as to the healing side of Tai Chi.

Tai Chi is seen by many as one of the best of the modern day 'stress-busters'. If you are suffering from stress, your body will behave in various negative ways. Examples of these are shallow breathing and stooped posture. If your body has this reaction, then it will actually make you feel more stressed. As you can see, a vicious circle soon starts. Tai Chi can help you to break that vicious circle.

Another way that Tai Chi is helpful for stress sufferers is that it takes you out of the stress environment. Whether you are going to a lesson or practising in your own back yard, you have physically and mentally removed yourself from the source of your stress and you will respond positively to that. Structural problems are one of the hidden causes of many illnesses. With so many people working long hours on equipment that is not ergonomically sound, the problem is widespread and getting worse. The close attention that Tai Chi pays to body alignment can help you with this sort of problem.

Many mental problems can be from a feeling of wanting to strive for something 'higher', but not quite knowing what it is. The aspect of Tai Chi that addresses 'Raising the Spirit', and building one's Chi can be an antidote to these feelings.

The side of Tai Chi that is concerned with energy development is no modern trend. It has evolved and been perfected over hundreds of years. Energy is per-

Examples of some of the many lines of energy (meridians) that run through the body.

ceived by the sensitive to be running in channels or 'meridians'. If these energy meridians are unobstructed, then the energy can flow easily. If there is a restriction of blockage then an energy imbalance can occur which can lead to sickness.

Also, we have spoken about Yin and Yang within your body. If there is not a good balance between Yin and Yang, then illness will result. Tai Chi addresses this aspect directly by cultivating your internal energy, or Chi, and distributing it evenly throughout the meridian systems.

This is the reason why many advanced Tai Chi practitioners learn healing arts such as Shiatsu. The healing side of the Tai Chi will then make a Yin Yang pair with the martial art side of the art.

Many people who learn Tai Chi to an advanced stage also study healing arts, such as Shiatsu. This forms a perfect Yin Yang pair with the martial side of Tai Chi.

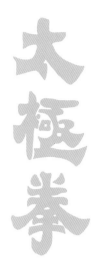

1

2

3

THE TEN ESSENCES OF TAI CHI

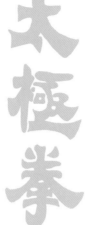

In Tai Chi, there are many formulas and ways towards better practice. These have come from the different Masters and experts who have taught the art through the years. The set of rules that I use is called the 'Ten Essences'.

Write them down and learn them. When you can reason your way through the Ten Essences, your Tai Chi will improve.

They were taught to me by my teacher, Christopher Pei, who has taken the Ten Essences as written by Yang Chengfu who arranged them into a logical sequence. The outcome of this is a sequence of rules or 'Essences' that capture the very heart of what Tai Chi is about. If you are ever unsure about anything in Tai Chi, always refer back to the Ten Essences. If you cannot resolve it in terms of the Essences as you understand them, it is time to ask your teacher or other authority in the subject. If you question Tai Chi in this way, you are on the path to understanding it.

THE TEN ESSENCES ARE:

1 Lift the head to raise the spirit

2 Lower the shoulders to sink the elbows

3 Curve the back and soften the chest

4 Loosen the waist

5 Separate the substantial from the insubstantial

6 Co-ordinate the upper and lower body

7 Continuity in movement

8 Unite mind with body

9 Use mind and not force

10 Seek stillness in motion and motion within stillness

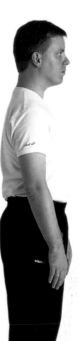

1. Lift the head to raise the spirit

This is the number one Essence, both in the sequence and in importance. If your posture is stooped or you are looking down all the time, you cannot lift your spirit. We all know the phrase 'walk tall'.

It is true in Tai Chi and life in general. If your head is up, then your spirit rises and you become stronger inside.

If you ever watch a Tai Chi Master, it will seem as if they are able to look at every individual person in the room. This is because the first essence is in place and they have a strong spirit.

6. Co-ordinate the upper and lower body

When you have understood the idea of double weight, you will start to examine other co-ordinations. The next thing to look at is whether your upper body is working in time with your lower body. If your legs finish a push before your arms, there is no upper and lower body co-ordination.

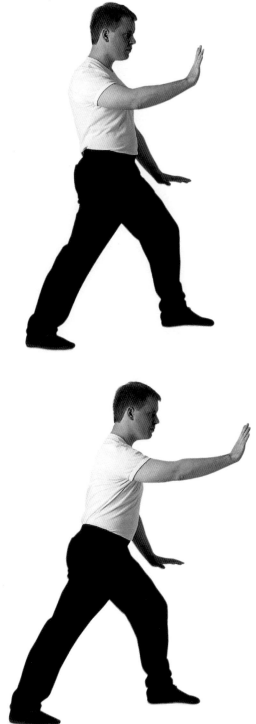

7. Continuity in movement

When your upper and lower body are co-ordinated, your movement will naturally become continuous. If your arms or legs stop at any point, then check your co-ordinations. The Tai Chi movement should be one continuous flow.

8. Unite mind with body

If your Tai Chi movement has become continuous, you then need to co-ordinate what you understand about the applications with the movements. If the intent of your mind is co-ordinated with your Tai Chi frame, you will understand this.

9. Use mind and not force

At this stage, you will have learned how to co-ordinate your intent with the movement. Energy is moved by intent, so when you can unify your intent with your body, you can unify your Energy with your intent. This is how you use mind instead of force.

10. Seek stillness in motion and motion within stillness

This is a very high level of Tai Chi. It means that you can perform all of the co-ordinations in the Ten Essences and not have to send your systems into overload trying to remember it all. It is the same as watching a master craftsman working alongside his apprentice. They may be doing the same job, but the Master will seem effortless in his endeavours.

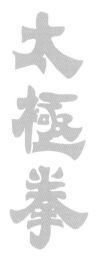

The Ten Essences should be worked through one after the other, as they flow into each other. You will soon get glimpses of what the higher essences are all about, but your practice will be more efficient if you work through the essences.

When you have reached the tenth essence, you start again at the first essence — Spirit. The difference is that this time around, the first essence will mean different things to you than it did the first time.

PREPARING YOUR BODY FOR TAI CHI

Most Tai Chi teachers have a sequence of warm-up exercises that they use to start their classes. The warm-up sequences that are used will vary from teacher to teacher, but there is usually a certain flavour to the movements that subtly defines them as Tai Chi exercises.

This raises an interesting point. If it is possible to perceive a difference between Tai Chi warm-up exercises and other warm-up exercises, then what is this difference?

The answer lies in the fact that these exercises have evolved over many years and have originated from ideas that seek to integrate the energies of the body and mind. After a few weeks' practice with these exercises, you will start to be able to sense your own Chi. This is a result of the integration aspect of the exercises. This is an important reason why your warm-up exercises should be practised regularly if you want to improve your Tai Chi skill.

With most of the exercises, there is no specific number of repetitions to be performed. The reason for this is that the final decision should be up to you. If there is an exercise that you particularly like, then there is no reason why you should not practise it as much as you wish. Sometimes when your body is trying to heal itself, you will be drawn to what your body needs. If you develop a favourite exercise, then your body may be responding positively to the changes that it may cause. Conversely, if an exercise seems more like torture, then perhaps you should avoid that one for a while.

When you practice ANY warm-up exercises, you should take notice of what your body is telling you. If it hurts – stop. You should never inflict damage upon yourself in your training. Pain is usually your body's way of telling you to stop doing something. Ignore the messages at your own peril. Tai Chi warm-up exercises should never be rushed and should not suddenly stop.

If you follow these guidelines, you should be able to avoid injury. If you are in any doubt, consult your teacher or your doctor.

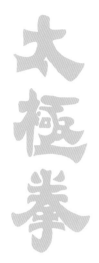

The Wu Chi position

The Wu Chi position will be explained more thoroughly in a later chapter. It is used in many of the warm-up exercises as a starting position. In the Wu Chi position, your feet are parallel, head up, shoulders down and arms relaxed. It should not take any real physical effort to hold the position, so you should be able to relax into the posture.

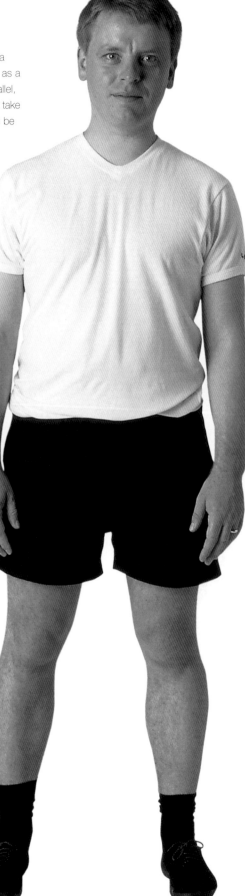

Warm-up exercises

1. Shaking and breathing

This exercise loosens and relaxes your body and is a good first exercise for your routine.

1 Start in the Wu Chi posture.

2 Begin by shaking your fingertips. This need not be particularly vigorous. It is designed to start bringing some movement into your body. Feel each individual fingertip as you shake. Make your inhalation and exhalation vigorous throughout the exercise.

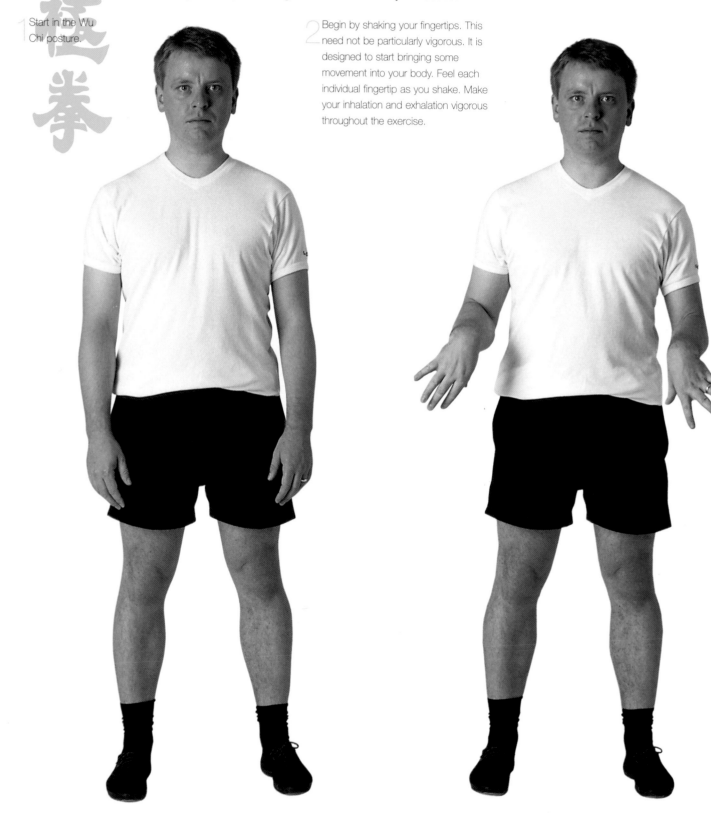

3 When you can 'feel into' each of your fingertips, move your attention further up your finger into the first joint. Let the joint becomes more relaxed. Carry on doing this exercise for all of the joints in your hand, working inward from your fingertips up to your wrist. Your hands should feel more relaxed by now.

4 Carry on with the exercise, gradually moving your attention from your wrist through to your forearm and elbow. Allow your elbow to loosen, and start to move the biceps and triceps muscles at the top of your arm. Finish by shaking your shoulders up and down, letting your arms hang free.

Allow the movement to gradually slow down and stop.

5 You now apply exactly the same exercise that you have just done with your arms, to your legs.

6 Put your weight into your left leg and start to shake the toes of your right leg

7 Gradually work through your toes, foot, ankle, lower leg, knee and thigh. You will also find that this is a good exercise for balancing on your standing leg.

Repeat the exercise for your left leg.

2. Swing your waist and arms

This exercise is another general exercise to loosen the whole of your body. It is also very good for releasing tension from your spine. A good mental image is to imagine a willow tree in a storm. The root is strong and will not move, but the upper half is flexible and free to move with the wind.

1 Stand in the Wu Chi posture.

2 Oscillate your waist to the left and the right. Whilst you are moving your waist, keep your body straight and your arms relaxed. Start quite slowly, but gradually build up speed. Do not become too vigorous with the movements, as this will make them difficult to control.

The lift for your arms comes from the rotation of your waist. As your waist rotates about an axis, a physical force lifts your arms. Do not just swing your arms, as this reduces the benefit of the exercise.

3 Your arms should swing around your waist. This gives a massage to your lower abdomen and the kidney area of your back.

When you have had enough, let your waist momentum gradually slow down and stop. Do not try to stop suddenly because this can lead to injury.

3. The Tai Chi Circle

This exercise teaches you how to breathe deeply and invigorate your body with a good supply of oxygen.

1 For this exercise, all of the breathing is done through your nose and your position remains stationary. Try to let your mind empty and keep your body relaxed. Stand with your feet parallel and one shoulder width apart. Look straight in front of you with your eyes relaxed. Turn your hands so that the palms face outward.

2 On an inward breath, raise both of your hands in a circle. Keep your shoulders down and synchronise the movement with your breathing.

3 When your hands reach the top of the circle, lower your shoulders and elbows.

4 Then press your palms down gently with the outward breath.

5 Start the movement again. Keep it as slow and relaxed as you can, so that your breathing deepens. When you become an expert at this exercise, you will be able to slow your breathing down so that it becomes deeper.

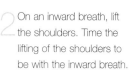

4. Shoulder rotations

It is important in any martial art to relax your shoulders. If your shoulders are stiff, then the rest of your body cannot relax and movement will be restricted.

2 On an inward breath, lift the shoulders. Time the lifting of the shoulders to be with the inward breath.

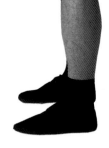

1 Start by standing in the Wu Chi position.

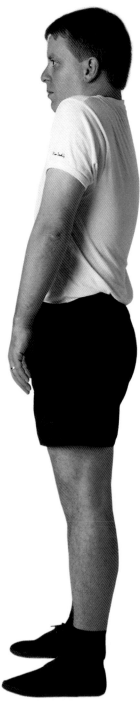

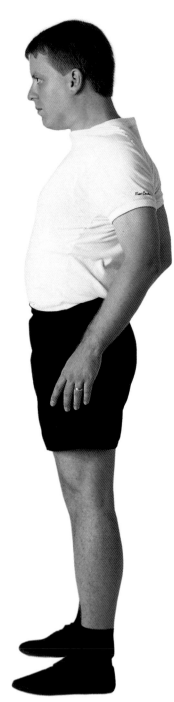

3 When your lungs are full and your shoulders are at their maximum, slowly allow your breath out and let your shoulders descend.

Repeat the movement several times, and then change the direction of shoulder rotation. Try to do the movement quite slowly, so that it is easier to time the movement of your shoulders with the movement of your breath.

5. Shoulder rotation with extended arms

This exercise is a more difficult version of the previous one. Attempt it only when you feel confident with the previous exercise.

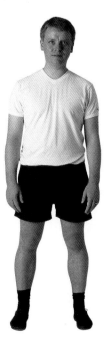

1 Start by standing in the Wu Chi position.

2 On an inward breath, imagine that your intake of air fills your arms, and let them float upwards until they are slightly lower than your shoulders.

3 Rotate your shoulders several times in both directions (the same way that you did for the last exercise). You will find that the exercise is made more difficult because your hands are raised. Try to keep them in the same position, but do not lock your shoulder joint.

It normally takes many years of practice before you can perform the exercise without moving your hands at all.

太極拳

6. Windmills

You will be able to develop your skill more efficiently if your shoulders are loose. This is the last sequence that will focus only on your shoulders.

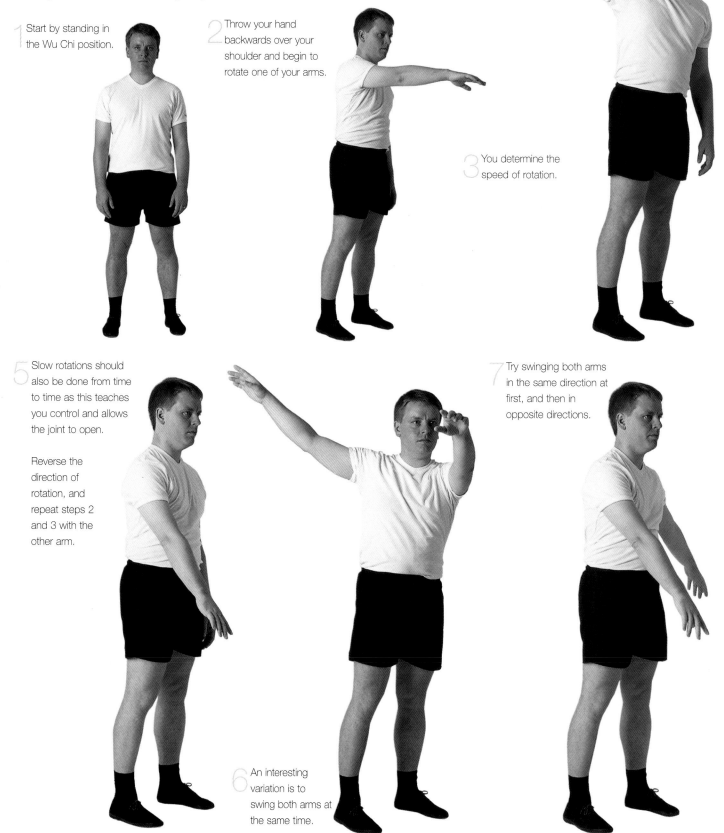

1 Start by standing in the Wu Chi position.

2 Throw your hand backwards over your shoulder and begin to rotate one of your arms.

3 You determine the speed of rotation.

5 Slow rotations should also be done from time to time as this teaches you control and allows the joint to open.

Reverse the direction of rotation, and repeat steps 2 and 3 with the other arm.

6 An interesting variation is to swing both arms at the same time.

7 Try swinging both arms in the same direction at first, and then in opposite directions.

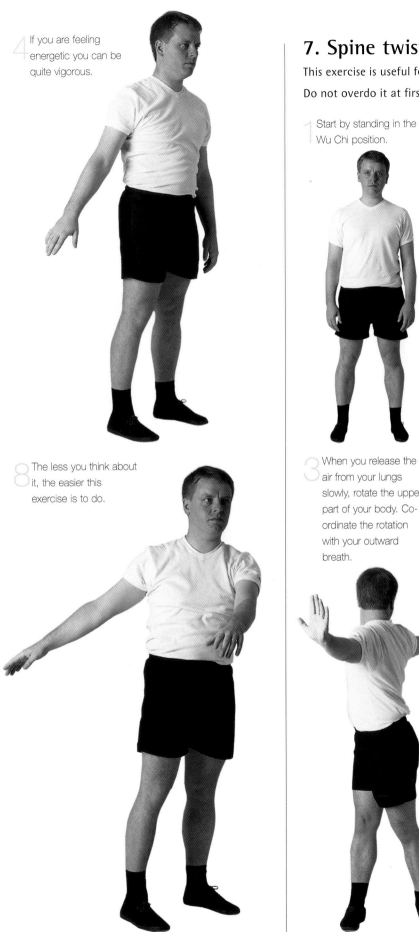

4 If you are feeling energetic you can be quite vigorous.

8 The less you think about it, the easier this exercise is to do.

7. Spine twist with your arms extended

This exercise is useful for unlocking your spine, keeping it healthy and supple. Do not overdo it at first and you will be on the way to a stronger back.

1 Start by standing in the Wu Chi position.

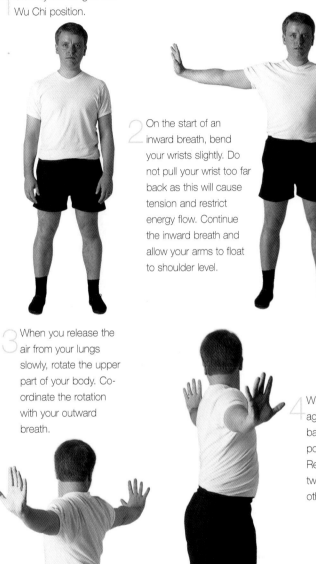

2 On the start of an inward breath, bend your wrists slightly. Do not pull your wrist too far back as this will cause tension and restrict energy flow. Continue the inward breath and allow your arms to float to shoulder level.

3 When you release the air from your lungs slowly, rotate the upper part of your body. Co-ordinate the rotation with your outward breath.

4 When you breathe in again, bring your body back to the central position in step 2. Repeat the exercise by twisting your body in the other direction.

Five or six repetitions will be enough at first. You may increase the amount as you become more supple.

Many people soon start to experience sensations in the centre of the palm. This is an important energy centre or *Tsubo*, the Japanese word for becoming active.

8. Waist rotations

Energy can become very 'locked up' in the pelvic area. This can lead to many problems in that region. This exercise teaches you to be more supple.

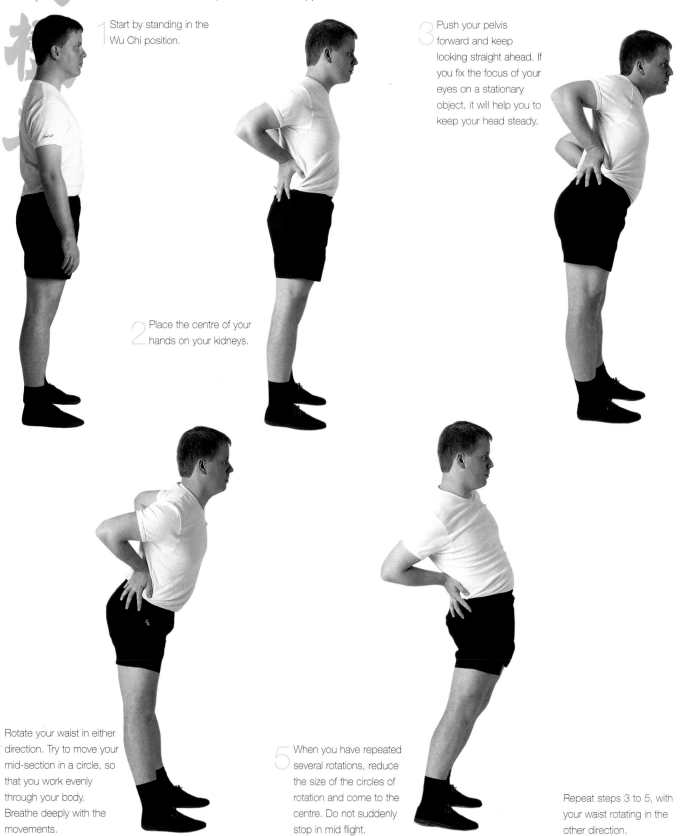

1 Start by standing in the Wu Chi position.

2 Place the centre of your hands on your kidneys.

3 Push your pelvis forward and keep looking straight ahead. If you fix the focus of your eyes on a stationary object, it will help you to keep your head steady.

4 Rotate your waist in either direction. Try to move your mid-section in a circle, so that you work evenly through your body. Breathe deeply with the movements.

5 When you have repeated several rotations, reduce the size of the circles of rotation and come to the centre. Do not suddenly stop in mid flight.

Repeat steps 3 to 5, with your waist rotating in the other direction.

9. Side push in horse-riding stance

This exercise helps balance the left and right sides of your body.

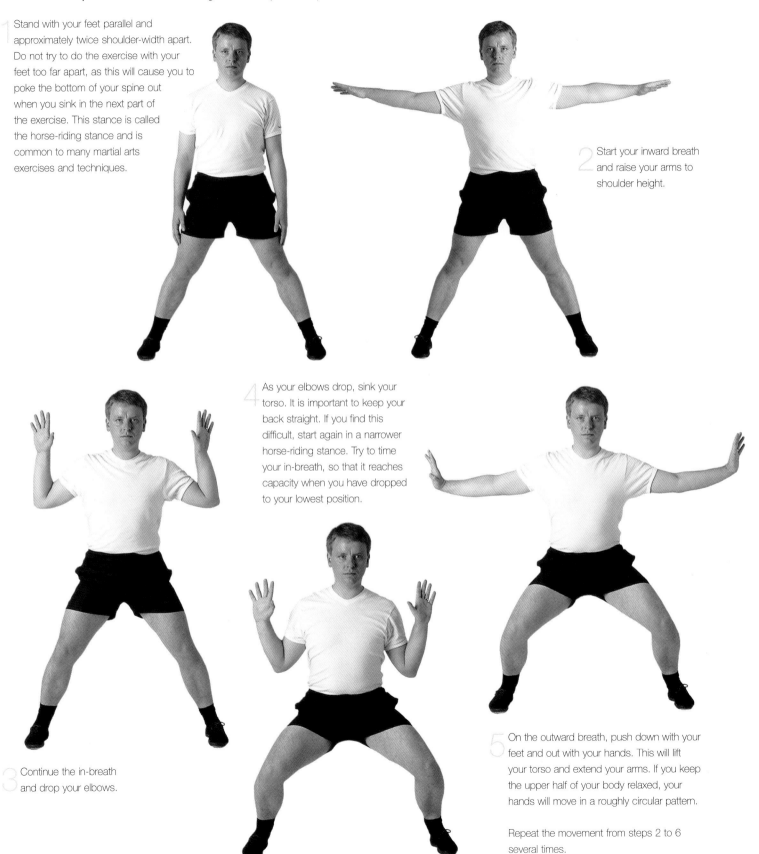

1 Stand with your feet parallel and approximately twice shoulder-width apart. Do not try to do the exercise with your feet too far apart, as this will cause you to poke the bottom of your spine out when you sink in the next part of the exercise. This stance is called the horse-riding stance and is common to many martial arts exercises and techniques.

2 Start your inward breath and raise your arms to shoulder height.

3 Continue the in-breath and drop your elbows.

4 As your elbows drop, sink your torso. It is important to keep your back straight. If you find this difficult, start again in a narrower horse-riding stance. Try to time your in-breath, so that it reaches capacity when you have dropped to your lowest position.

5 On the outward breath, push down with your feet and out with your hands. This will lift your torso and extend your arms. If you keep the upper half of your body relaxed, your hands will move in a roughly circular pattern.

Repeat the movement from steps 2 to 6 several times.

10. Side stretch in horse-riding stance

This stretch helps to keep the energy meridians in the side of the body healthy. This will help you to control the movements that you practise in your forms.

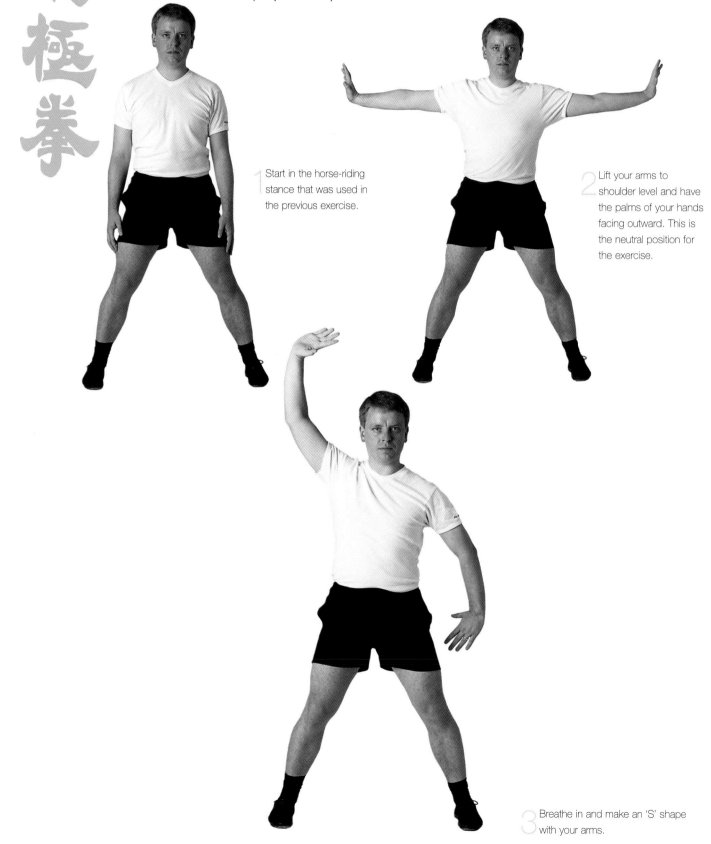

1 Start in the horse-riding stance that was used in the previous exercise.

2 Lift your arms to shoulder level and have the palms of your hands facing outward. This is the neutral position for the exercise.

3 Breathe in and make an 'S' shape with your arms.

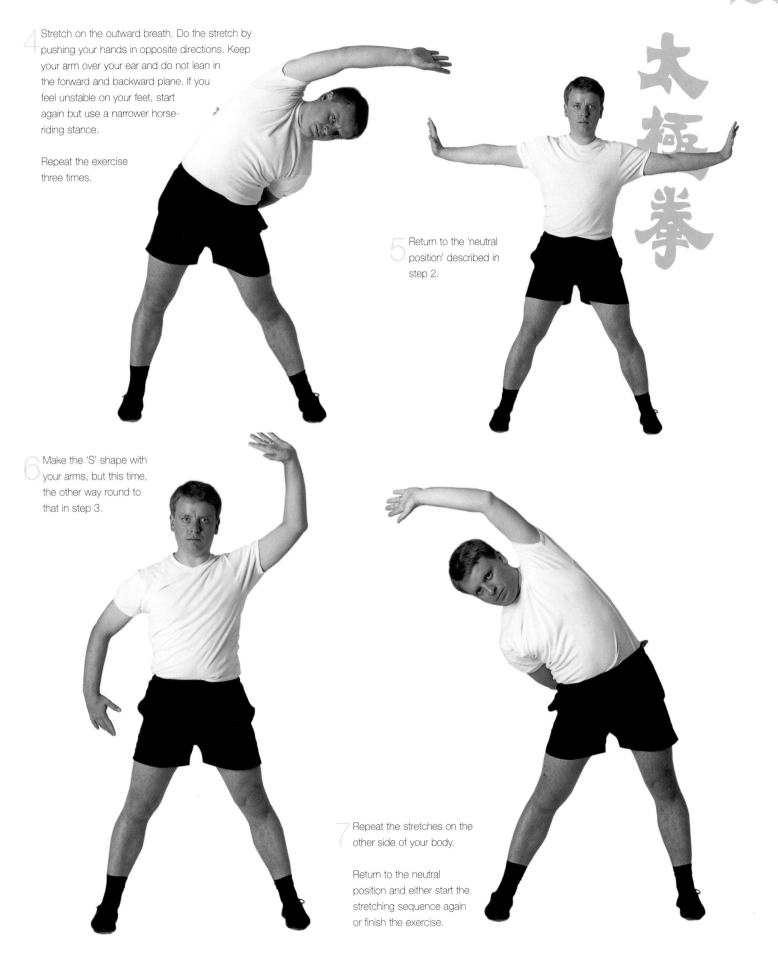

4 Stretch on the outward breath. Do the stretch by pushing your hands in opposite directions. Keep your arm over your ear and do not lean in the forward and backward plane. If you feel unstable on your feet, start again but use a narrower horse-riding stance.

Repeat the exercise three times.

5 Return to the 'neutral position' described in step 2.

6 Make the 'S' shape with your arms, but this time, the other way round to that in step 3.

7 Repeat the stretches on the other side of your body.

Return to the neutral position and either start the stretching sequence again or finish the exercise.

11. 'No spiders on the ceiling'

This exercise was taught to me by my first Tai Chi teacher who was a very talented Chinese gentleman. When we were practising the sequence he would call out, 'No spiders on the ceiling', at the part where you lean back. This was his humorous way of reminding us to not tilt our heads back and look at the ceiling, as this can cause injury. It has therefore become one of my favourite exercises because it always reminds me of my first teacher.

It is a very powerful exercise and is very good for keeping your spine healthy, as long as you do not strain yourself. If you cannot practise it comfortably, work with the other exercises for some time until your body has become more flexible.

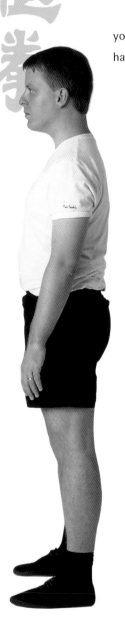

1 Start in the Wu Chi position.

2 Breathe in and lift your hands to shoulder level

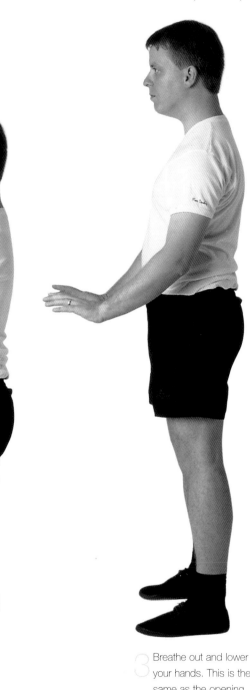

3 Breathe out and lower your hands. This is the same as the opening movement of the Tai Chi form.

太極拳

4 Breathe in, raise your arms and lean back. Keep your chin tucked in and look forward (remember – no spiders!). Your arms are in a circular shape as if you were holding a large beach ball. Do not lean back too far.

5 On the outward breath drop your body forward into a forward bend.

6 This should be quite relaxed. You do not need to try to stretch in this position, just let your spine release itself.

7 Bend your knees, so that you are in a squatting position. The work here is done with your legs. Avoid back strain by keeping it relaxed and in the same position. Let your legs make the effort.

8 Stand up by straightening your legs. Do not bend your back. If your arms are relaxed, your hands will naturally come together at the Tan Tien point on your abdomen.

Repeat the exercise from steps 1, 7, or finish.

12. Hip rotation

This exercise is particularly useful for any martial art that involves kicking, as it strengthens the hip joint in all planes of motion. It is also helpful if you want to improve your balance, as it is done on one leg.

1 Lift the knee of your right leg as high as you can.

2 Rotate the knee three times in a clockwise direction.

3 Rest for a while by placing your foot on the floor.

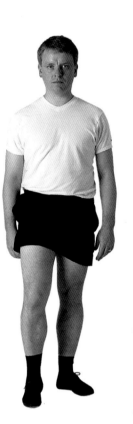

4 Lift your knee again and turn it in the opposite direction (anti-clockwise).

5 Rest your leg again.

6 Lift your knee again.

7 Push your heel in a forward circle, as though you were thrusting your foot out.

8 Rest your leg again. Now reverse the direction of the last turn, so that the motion is similar to stamping on the floor.

Repeat the exercise with your left leg. The easy way to remember the exercise is that you will rotate your knee in the forward, backward, clockwise and anti-clockwise directions.

If you find it difficult to balance, fix your eyes on a mark on the wall and try to keep the marker steady. This will help you to keep the upper half of your body steady.

When you can do the sequence without much effort, try doing it without putting your foot on the floor in between rotations. When this becomes easy, try increasing the number of rotations. This will normally take some time to achieve, as most people who have not done this exercise before find it quite strenuous. Do not compromise the exercise by doing it more quickly, as you will only be fooling yourself.

13. Knee rotation

This simple exercise can help you keep your knees healthy. Do not practise it if you have a knee problem, as it may simply make matters worse. Supple knees are vital to Tai Chi.

1 Stand with both feet together, ankles touching. Bend your knees slightly and reach down to rest the palms of your hands on your kneecaps.

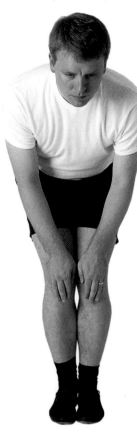

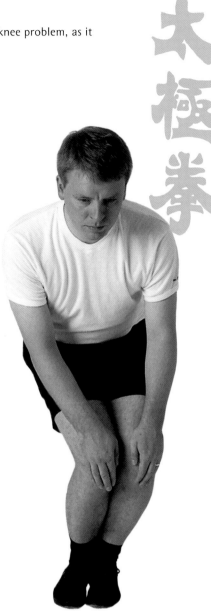

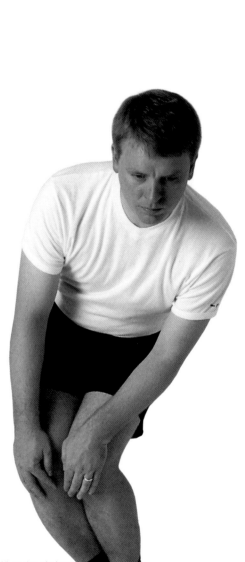

3 When you have made several circles in one direction, slow down and stop. Then repeat the exercise a similar number of times in the opposite direction.

2 Make small circles with the knees. Allow the circles to gradually increase in size. Do not try to make the knee circles too large (especially as a beginner) as this can strain the knee.

The exercise is performed with feet flat on the floor. You may feel that your balance is slightly wobbly in the beginning. This is improved by focusing your eyes on a point on the floor. The point should be static and approximately one metre (three feet) away. By now you should have the idea of how to keep your balance in an unusual position.

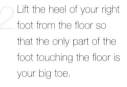

14. Ankle rotation

Your ankle joint has to carry more weight than any other joint in your body. If you have a problem with your ankle, it will be nearly impossible to keep your body straight because it is similar to trying to construct a building on loose foundations. If you have strong and supple ankles, your Tai Chi will improve and your posture has a better chance of improving.

1 Stand in the Wu Chi position.

2 Lift the heel of your right foot from the floor so that the only part of the foot touching the floor is your big toe.

3 Keep your leg relaxed and your toe in the same position on the floor. Rotate your knee in a clockwise direction. Start with small rotations and build up to larger ones. Keeping your toe fixed and your knee rotating will cause the most movement in the ankle.

4 After ten to twenty rotations, slow down to a stop. Repeat the exercise with an anti-clockwise rotation.

Repeat the exercise on the other leg.

Do not lean your body during the exercise. You will probably find that your standing leg has to work hard for this exercise. This is because it is carrying all of your weight. After you have completed the exercise, give your legs a good shake to loosen them up again.

15. Heel lifts

This exercise will teach you how to work with your calf muscles.

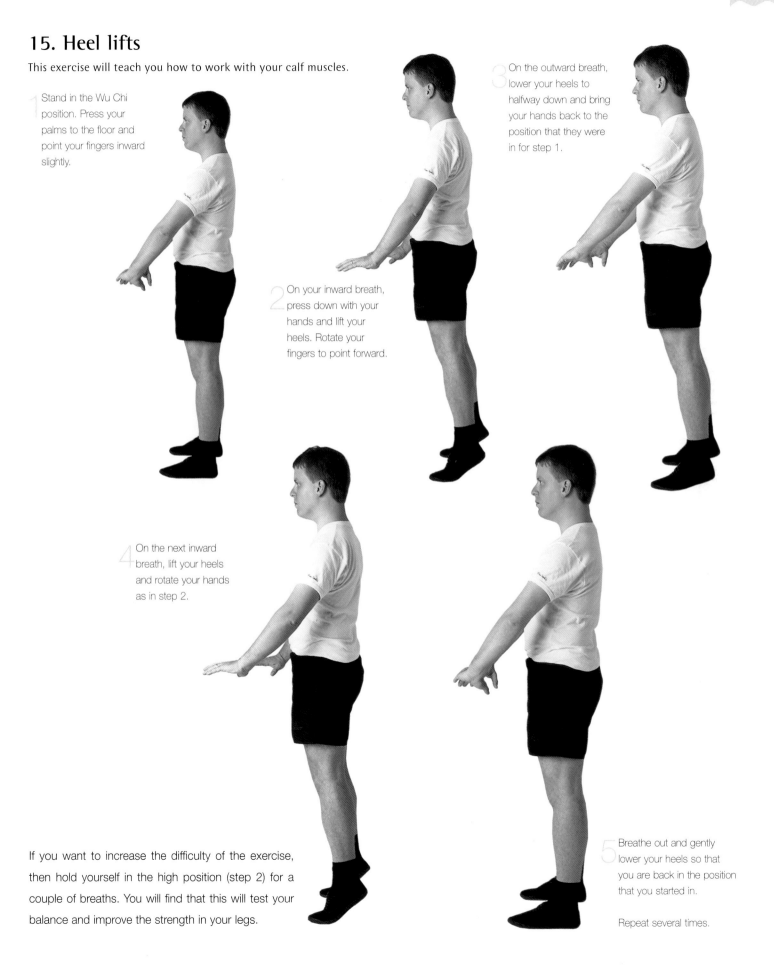

1 Stand in the Wu Chi position. Press your palms to the floor and point your fingers inward slightly.

2 On your inward breath, press down with your hands and lift your heels. Rotate your fingers to point forward.

3 On the outward breath, lower your heels to halfway down and bring your hands back to the position that they were in for step 1.

4 On the next inward breath, lift your heels and rotate your hands as in step 2.

5 Breathe out and gently lower your heels so that you are back in the position that you started in.

Repeat several times.

If you want to increase the difficulty of the exercise, then hold yourself in the high position (step 2) for a couple of breaths. You will find that this will test your balance and improve the strength in your legs.

16. Ankle jumps

This slightly comical-looking exercise is very good for improving your co-ordination and keeping your upper body relaxed. If you find that the exercise makes you laugh, you have discovered another secret of relaxation!

1 Start with your feet together and your arms relaxed.

2 On an outward breath push up from the floor with your ankle. It is important that you land with the toe first, as you will be able to break your fall. If you come down with your heel first, you will send a shock wave through your body that may cause injury.

You should aim to make as little noise as possible when you land. This teaches you how to absorb the impact of landing. If your arms are relaxed, they will move with your body. If your arms are stiff, it will be very difficult to get off the ground.

The height that you jump is relatively unimportant. It will improve as you get better at the exercise. It is more important to land softly and keep your body relaxed. You will also notice that the movement requires a very fast breath. It would be very difficult to slow the breathing down for this exercise.

17. Ankle jumps with rocking

This exercise is simply a different way of doing the last exercise. It works your muscles in a different way and continues to develop your leg muscles. If you want to make your ankle jumps more difficult, try doing them on the beach. It is more difficult to take off if you are standing on sand.

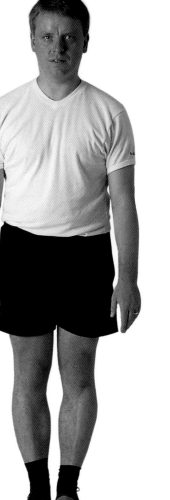

1 Start with your feet together and your arms relaxed.

2 Lift the balls of your feet from the floor.

3 Rock forward onto the front of your feet and use the momentum to assist your jump. Remember to be careful how you land.

18. Swimming Dragon

This exercise is good for stretching your legs and working your lungs. Work equally on both sides and do not try dropping your body too low, as you may strain your muscles and you will lose control of the exercise.

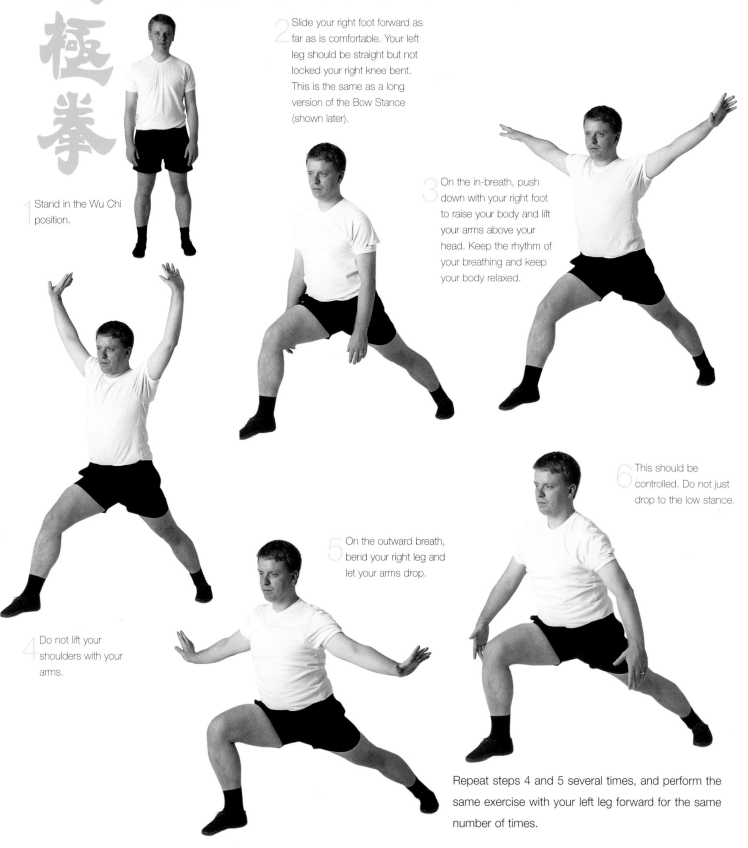

2 Slide your right foot forward as far as is comfortable. Your left leg should be straight but not locked your right knee bent. This is the same as a long version of the Bow Stance (shown later).

3 On the in-breath, push down with your right foot to raise your body and lift your arms above your head. Keep the rhythm of your breathing and keep your body relaxed.

1 Stand in the Wu Chi position.

6 This should be controlled. Do not just drop to the low stance.

5 On the outward breath, bend your right leg and let your arms drop.

4 Do not lift your shoulders with your arms.

Repeat steps 4 and 5 several times, and perform the same exercise with your left leg forward for the same number of times.

19. Candlestick

When you perform this exercise, you can imagine that your head and torso form a candlestick. If you lean over in any direction, you will loose the candle. The image is simply a way of reminding you to keep your back straight and your head up. The exercise has a quite powerful stretch on your legs, so it is advisable to be fairly well warmed-up before you start it.

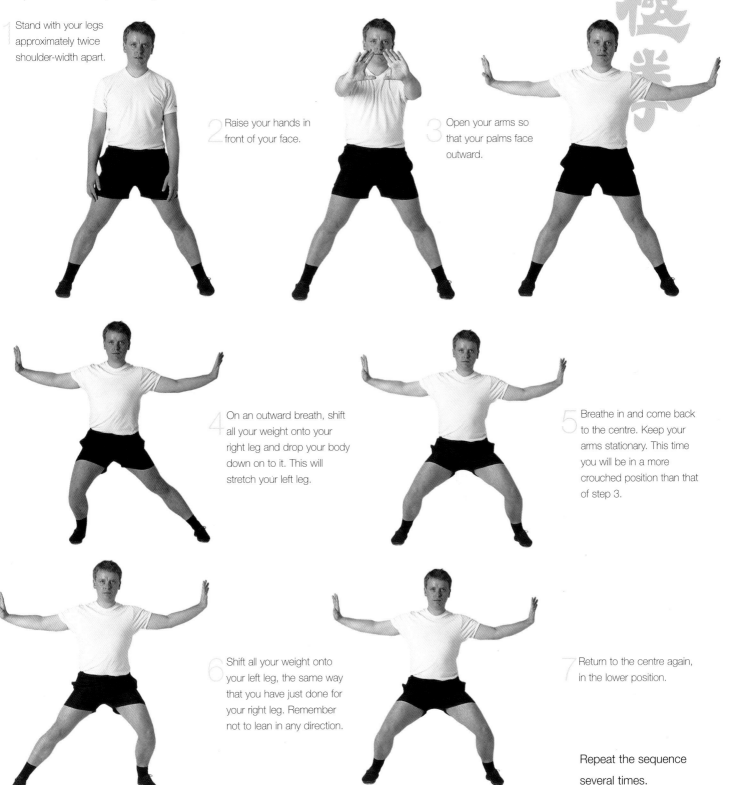

1 Stand with your legs approximately twice shoulder-width apart.

2 Raise your hands in front of your face.

3 Open your arms so that your palms face outward.

4 On an outward breath, shift all your weight onto your right leg and drop your body down on to it. This will stretch your left leg.

5 Breathe in and come back to the centre. Keep your arms stationary. This time you will be in a more crouched position than that of step 3.

6 Shift all your weight onto your left leg, the same way that you have just done for your right leg. Remember not to lean in any direction.

7 Return to the centre again, in the lower position.

Repeat the sequence several times.

20. Wine glass

This exercise is excellent for opening the meridians in the sides of you body. The visualisation is that you should imagine you are balancing a wine glass on the palm of your hand, and do not want to spill a drop. When you have become proficient with the exercise, you will actually be able to do the exercise with a drink resting on your palm. It makes a good party trick, especially when other people think that they can also do it!

1 Start in the Wu Chi position.

2 Push your right leg forward so that you are in the Bow Stance. Raise your right hand and imagine that you have a glass of wine balancing on it.

3 Shift your weight back onto your left leg and point your fingers inward.

4 Continue the path with your right hand as you sink down slightly further.

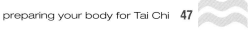

5 Begin to shift your weight forward on to your right leg, and continue moving your hand round.

6 With your weight fully on your right leg, continue to raise your arm, keeping the palm flat.

7 Shift your weight again onto your left leg and arch your back slightly. Look up to your hand, which should be above your face.

8 Begin to push your weight back onto your right leg and allow your hand to come back to the position it was in for step 2.

9 Try to make the movement smooth and continuous.

Repeat steps 2 to 7 several times. Perform the exercise again on the left side of your body, the same number of times.

10 If you are feeling adventurous, try it with both hands moving and your feet in the Wu Chi position.

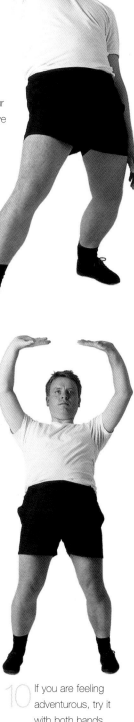

太極拳

PREPARING YOUR MIND FOR TAI CHI

Meditation has always been associated with Tai Chi. Some regard the importance of meditation in Tai Chi as one of the defining factors as to what Tai Chi actually is. The word 'meditation', often conjures up an image of Buddha or a yoga student sitting in the lotus position. Whilst this style of quiet meditation is perfectly valid, meditation need not be limited to this idea. Indeed, the Tai Chi form itself is a form of meditation when done correctly.

Buddha is a common image that comes to mind when people think about meditation.

Why is meditation a useful aspect of Tai Chi training? Try and think of an answer yourself before continuing. There are so many different ways of looking at it that you will stand a good chance of coming up with a reasonable answer.

When we are in our busy work routines it can feel as if our minds have a momentum of their own. We charge from one task to the next without even a second thought. This certainly gets the job done, but what about when the job is finished? Your mind can sometimes continue racing. If there is no immediate task, random thoughts can seem to come from nowhere. If you wish to learn how to relax your mind, you need to learn how to control these thoughts. The first meditation exercise helps you learn this skill.

If you have worked yourself into the state where it feels like your mind and body are separate entities, you have started to harm yourself. As you become more stressed your body and mind become separate and relaxation becomes difficult. The second meditation exercise will help you with this aspect.

In order to develop your sense of Chi, you will need to use your imagination to open the routes and let your Chi follow your intent. The final meditation, the 'Microcosmic Orbit' teaches you how this is done.

Meditation Exercise 1

This exercise can be done at any time when you have a couple of minutes to yourself. It is also useful to quieten the mind before the next two meditations. You can be in any position, and many find it easier with eyes closed, but this is not vital for the exercise.

The exercise involves remaining quiet and counting slowly from one to ten in your mind. If anything at all interrupts your consciousness, such as a stray thought, the awareness of a noise or even the sound of your own breathing, you must start again.

If you can make it to a count of three, your concentration is very good. If you can make it to ten, then you should probably be reading a more advanced book than this one!

It is also a useful exercise to remember if you lose your concentration during form practice.

太極拳

Meditation Exercise 2

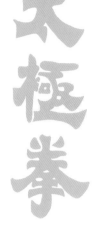

Choose the correct environment. Make sure you are in a well-ventilated room with plenty of fresh air. Keep warm, as the temperature of your body will drop during meditation, so you may wish to put more clothes on. Switch on the answer-phone if you have one. Try to minimise any disturbances for the next twenty minutes or so. Sometime you may enjoy burning essential oils or listening to soft music. This can enhance the mood for meditation.

1 Choose either a sitting or lying down position. Close your eyes and relax. Have your mouth gently closed but do not clench your jaw. Breathe through your nose. Focus your mind on your breathing and let it become soft and deep. Spend a few minutes simply focusing your attention on your breathing, allowing it to become soft and regular.

2 Bring your attention to your forehead. Relax the muscles and skin on your forehead. Do this by imagining that every time you breathe out, the tension is just falling away. Do the same for your eyes and the muscles of your face.

3 Work down through your body relaxing your neck, shoulders, arms, chest, abdomen, waist, thighs, knees, lower leg, ankles and feet. When your attention reaches your feet, pause for a while by bringing your attention back to your breathing. Make sure that your breathing is still relaxed, deep and regular.

4 Now bring your attention back to your forehead. Instead of relaxing the outer skin and muscles, work with your attention slightly deeper within your body. Every that time you go through your body you are relaxing it with the intent of your mind. This allows you to 'peel off' layers of tension rather like the layers of an onion skin.

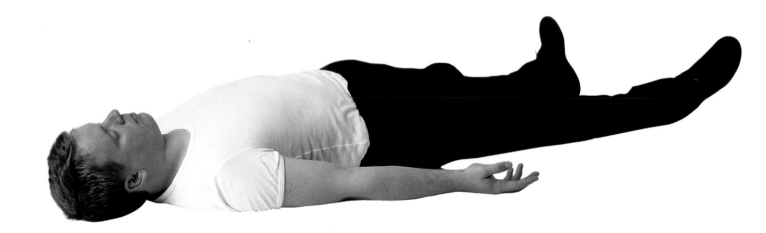

Meditation Exercise 3 - the Microcosmic Orbit

This meditation circulates energy around two meridians called the Governing Vessel and the Conception Vessel. The Governing Vessel runs up your spine from your perineum and loops over the top of your skull to the roof of your mouth. The Conception Vessel runs from the tip of your tongue to join with the Governing Vessel at your perineum.

1 The idea is to circulate energy through the two meridians in a circuit. The circuit needs to be completed by placing your tongue on the roof of your mouth. Your tongue should be on the roof of your mouth for form practice for exactly the same reason.

The meditation can be done in a sitting or lying down position. My preference is a sitting position as it is more difficult to accidentally fall asleep.

2 Warm-up' your mind for the meditation with one of the earlier meditation exercises. Your mind should be quite still and relaxed.

Use your imagination to create a channel of energy that starts at your perineum. Next, take it to a point in between your kidneys (the Ming Men point). Imagine that the energy travels in a straight path to the point in between your shoulder blades. Carry on up your spine to a point at the base of your skull.

3 Take your imagination and intent around your skull to the topmost point. This is the Crown Point. Take your intent from that point, through the centre of your forehead over your nose and to the roof of your mouth.

4 The energy then travels through your tongue and down the centre of your windpipe. Carry on through your breastbone and down to your navel. Just below your navel is another important energy point called the Tan Tien. This will become the focus point of your movement when your Tai Chi becomes more advanced. Finish the cycle by taking the energy through your groin and back to your perineum to start again.

5 When you become accustomed to the meditation, you will sense the energy rather than just using your imagination. This is the part that most people try to rush. If you relax more and let things take their own speed, it will actually happen faster than if you try to rush the process.

6 When you have finished meditation, bring yourself out of the state slowly. If you have been deeply relaxed, you should not suddenly try to jolt back to normal consciousness.

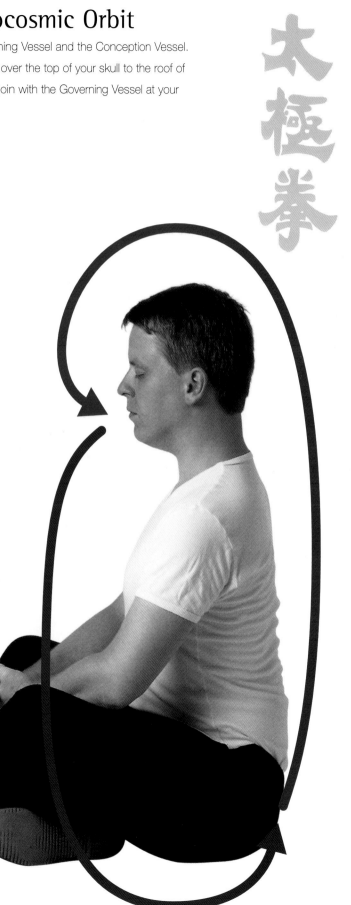

JOINING YOUR BODY AND MIND

Correct breathing

Do you know how you breathe? This seems like a stupid question. Of course you know how to breathe. Breathing is, however, an important part of Tai Chi exercise as it is with many other systems such as yoga. Obviously, there is a little more to it than just sitting there breathing. Before you read further, try the following exercise – you can stay sitting down for this.

1 Place the palms of both of your hands flat over your Tan Tien point (just below the navel).

2 Take a big deep breath.

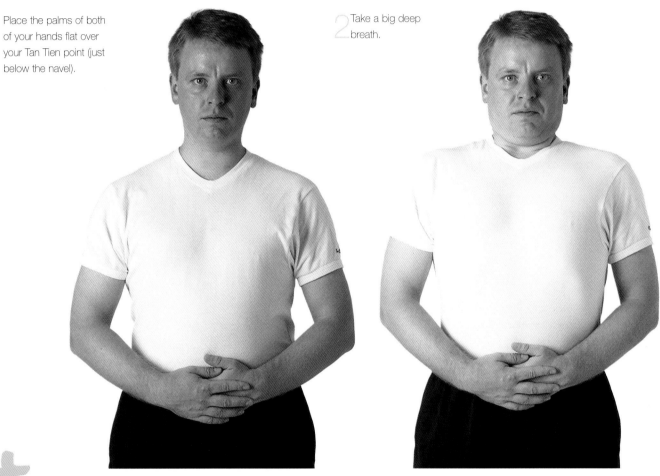

Did your abdomen lift your hands as you breathed in? If so, then you are practising abdominal breathing or 'breathing from the Tan Tien' , which is essential to Tai Chi. If, like many others, you found that most of the movement was from the chest area then you need to examine your breathing.

One of the reasons that people 'chest breathe' is connected to the well-known 'fight or flight' syndrome. The idea is that in an emergency situation, the fight or flight reflex takes over. One of the many effects is that your breathing becomes quicker and shallower. This is your body's effort to get as much oxygen into the system as possible in a short amount of time.

When your body is in this mode, certain functions will be restricted or stopped completely. These will be the ones that have no use in this panic reaction. Examples of these are making love, digestion and natural relaxation. This makes sense. The primal survival instinct would not work well if you felt the urge to fall asleep when you were under attack!

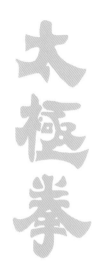

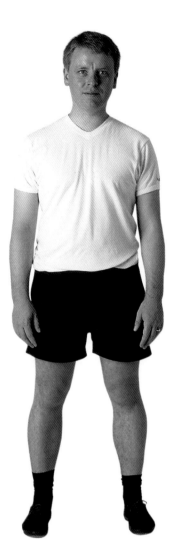

imagine that you are breathing from your Tan Tien. This movement of the Tan Tien will move your diaphragm in a way that aids natural breathing.

Repeat the exercise from the beginning of this section, but this time try to alter your breathing pattern so that your Tan Tien moves out when you breathe in. Place your hands on the Tan Tien so that you can see and feel the movement better. Notice how you can breathe more deeply and get more air in to your lungs if you breathe like this.

This is the preferred way of breathing in Tai Chi and most Chi Gung forms. If you find it difficult, do not worry. Never force your breathing into this pattern. As your Tai Chi skill level increases, your body will make the changes that make this kind of breathing possible. If you try to force it into your movement before you are ready, you will cause more harm than good. Practise it in your relaxation exercises and it will gradually work itself into your Tai Chi.

In our modern lives, many people are stuck halfway between the panic mode and the relaxed mode. This is partly because the fight or flight system is not usually appropriate in our modern lives. For example, the adrenaline response when you are 'cut-up' on the motorway may get you 'revved up', but you cannot use the energy. This often means that you never really come out of the panic mode and many of the functions that need the relaxed mode will be impaired.

This can also have an effect on your body posture. It requires very little imagination to see that different muscles and support systems will develop if you are constantly chest breathing rather than abdominal breathing.

Athletes and singers also know this secret. In their training they are frequently told to 'breathe from the diaphragm'. This is the correct idea, but can you really imagine your own diaphragm? It is normally easier to

You need to stand correctly and breathe correctly for your body to be balanced, allowing the energies to flow freely.

As you become more skilled in Tai Chi, your breathing will alter. You should never push your body into something it is not yet ready for. Allow your body to dictate the pace.

Standing exercises

太極拳

Standing exercises have been a part of traditional Chinese martial arts training for many years. They have been widely used to fight illness in the sick and increase strength and stamina in the healthy.

These exercises and others like them were the basis from which the Taoist monks practised the energy-building that eventually became Tai Chi as we know it. The exercises work directly with improving your posture and helping you to unlock your own energy. In the old days of martial arts schools in China, a master would make their students hold one of the standing exercises for the time it takes an incense stick to burn before they would teach them their skill. If you try to hold one of these positions for more than a few minutes, you will understand the high level that the masters demanded before the student could even start.

The following five exercises are from a system called 'Zhan Zhuang', or 'standing like a tree'. The first one, the Wu Chi position, is not physically demanding but you may find it difficult if you are constantly on the go in your normal life. The other exercises are more physically strenuous in different ways. Practise them all, and when you can manage them all individually for fifteen minutes, try the sequence. This will have taught you how to strengthen your posture and move your own Chi.

1. The Wu Chi position

The Wu Chi position has already been mentioned as a starting place for some of the Tai Chi exercises and the beginning of the forms. Wu Chi is symbolic of the beginning of the Universe, before Yin and Yang came into play. The Taoist idea is that from nothing – Wu Chi – the forces of Yin and Yang began to separate and divide. From the two primal forces, Yin and Yang, the whole of the Universe was made. This is also symbolised in the start of the form beginning with Wu Chi. The opening move represents the creation of Yin and Yang and the movements of the form represent the Universe.

Standing in Wu Chi for a period of time is not as easy as it looks for most people. The fact that you are doing nothing tends to go against the grain for somebody who has actually got out of his or her chair and has the intent to exercise. My advice is just to try it. You may find it nearly drives you crazy, just standing there doing nothing. This is a sign that you need to take control of your energy. If you can stand in Wu Chi for ten minutes or so, then you will be ready for the next standing exercises. Do not forget that by practising Wu Chi you are in the position of primal energy – which is a very good place to start.

To get into the Wu Chi position, stand with your feet shoulder width apart and parallel. Let your arms hang loose and do not pull your shoulders back and let them sink. Lift the crown of your head and feel your feet pushing into the floor. This will open your spine. Remember not to lock your knees. Slow your breathing and let it drop to the Tan Tien. As your breathing becomes deeper, your mind will become quieter. Feel your energy grounding itself through your feet and your spirit lifting through the crown of your head.

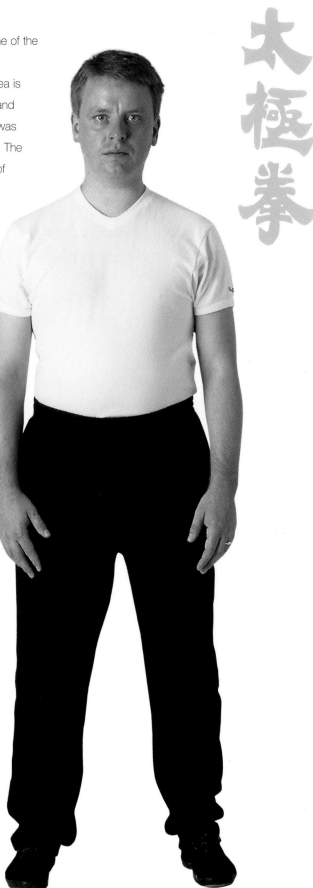

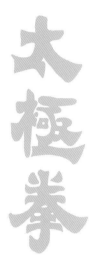

2. Holding a Balloon

When you can stand in Wu Chi for ten to fifteen minutes comfortably, you can move to the next exercise. This is the progression that you will take through the exercises until you can perform them all in a cycle. This exercise starts in the Wu Chi position but is more advanced. You will probably feel as if you are starting again with your training. This is a good sign that you are moving forward.

Start in the Wu Chi position. Bend your knees slightly but keep your back straight. It should feel as if you were sitting on the edge of a chair but keeping the weight in your legs. You will feel your thigh muscles being worked. If you are not sure about your back alignment, stand against a wall at first so that you can build an internal reference. Raise your arms. You should imagine that you are holding a three-dimensional balloon in your arms. Do not squash it against your chest. Your arm position is the same as 'Ward-off', a position that you will learn later in the Tai Chi form.

3. Holding your Belly

This exercise will seem easy after the last one. It helps you to focus energy into your Tan Tien and moves your energy in a downward direction and thus grounds it for you.

Start from the second position, holding the balloon. Drop your arms to a lower position. Be aware of any internal changes that happen during or after this transition.

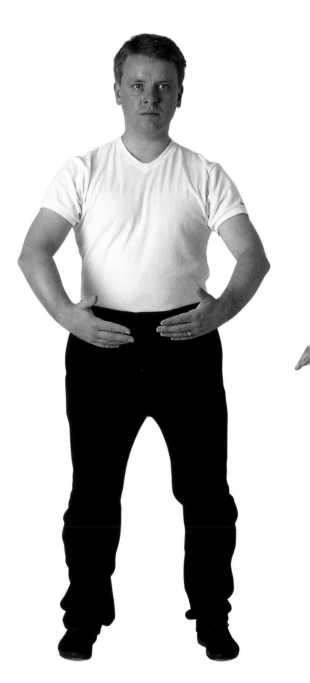

4. Standing in a Stream

This exercise will teach you another way of working your energy. Again, the energy is directed downwards and is therefore useful for grounding.

Start in the Wu Chi position. Turn your hands outwards and press down. Imagine that you are standing in a stream of running water and that you need to sink your weigh to stop it from washing you away. Imagine that your arms are resisting their natural buoyancy in the water.

5. Raising your Arms

This is the most demanding of all the standing positions because your arms are in an elevated position. In this position, the meridians that correspond to the fire element are opened. Practising this exercise properly will increase your inner core energy that helps you to define yourself. Fire energy is also connected to your creative abilities.

To do this exercise properly, you need to be able to relax into it. If you try it before you are ready, it will cause too much tension to be able to work properly.

Start in the second position, holding the balloon. Raise and rotate your arms.

The full cycle

The next logical step after you have learned to stand in all the positions is to do them one after the other. This is an advanced way of practising but will cause no harm as long as you do not try to do too much too quickly. Some teachers place great importance upon the sequence. In my lesson, I regard it as more important to work in a way that feels right for you. It is a good idea to start with the Wu Chi position and finish with a couple of minutes simply standing in it.

I have also found people who really do not like this way of training. If you are one of these, do not feel that you cannot learn Tai Chi – remember these exercises are only a part of a much bigger entity of which Tai Chi is another part.

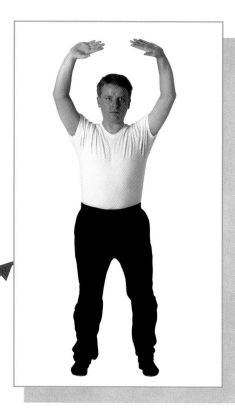

5. Raising your Arms

4. Standing in a Stream

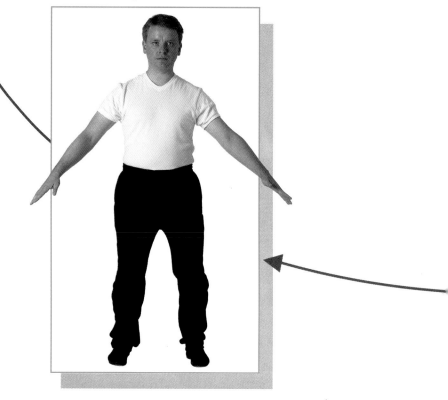

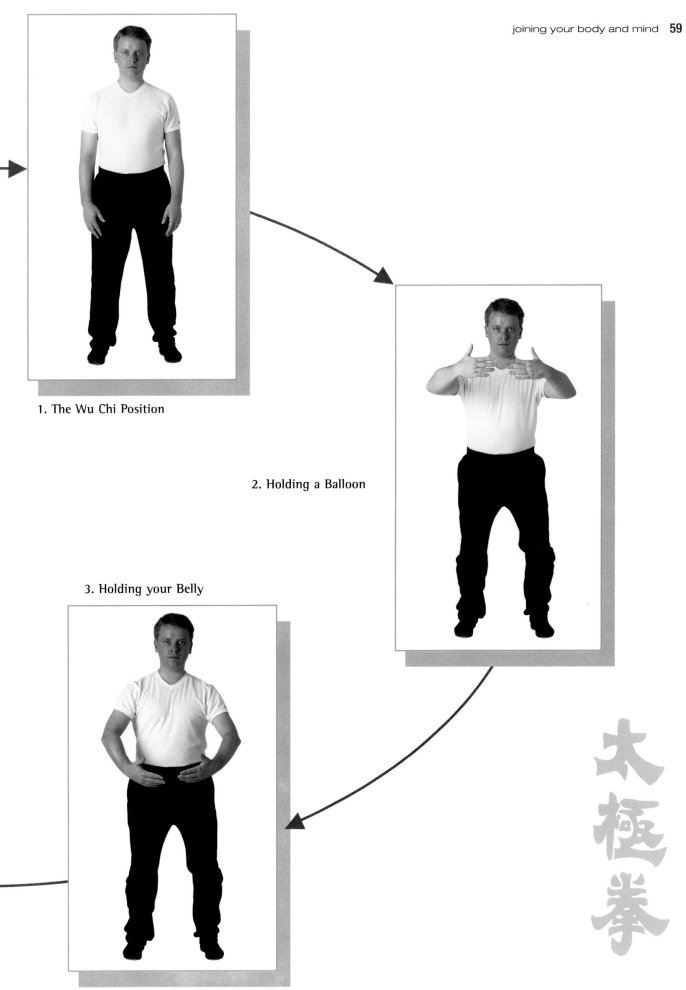

1. The Wu Chi Position

2. Holding a Balloon

3. Holding your Belly

UNDERSTANDING TAI CHI FORMS

When you think of what Tai Chi actually is, there is normally a mental image of somebody moving gracefully through a set of movements. This set of movements is usually called the Tai Chi form. Every style of Tai Chi, whether it is one of the older and more traditional ones, or one of the later adaptations, will have its own form. This is an aspect that Tai Chi shares with many other martial arts. For example, external styles such as karate and Tae Kwon Do consider pattern practice as being vital to the routine. In karate, forms or 'kata' are regarded as being the heart of the technique.

Why are Tai Chi forms so important?

The reason is that all of the information that you need to know about your style is contained within the form. This can lead to a common, but incorrect, assumption - that if all the information that you need is within the form, then form practice alone is all that you need.

Although form practice is unquestionably important in Tai Chi, you will not reach an advanced level if you only practise form. You will also need other aspects such as energy-building and working with other people. You cannot learn a martial art if you do not know what it is like to push someone or to be pushed? The same is also true of karate training. It would be impossible to imagine a karate student ('karateka') who has never tried sparring or destruction techniques.

In karate, the 'kata' is the equivalent of the 'form'. It is considered to be the heart of the style.

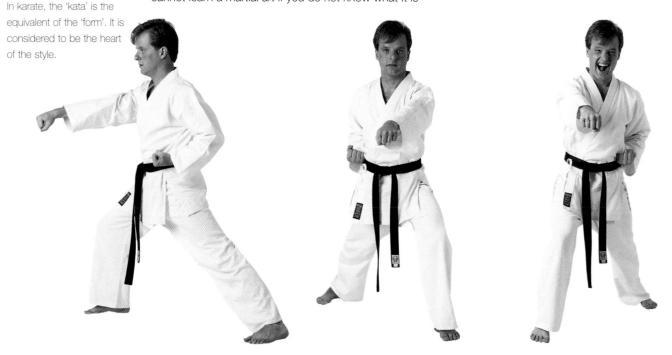

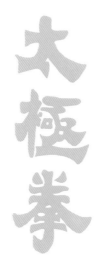

Forms work your body in different ways. For example, the movement of White Crane Spreads its Wings will test you in an entirely different way to Brush Knee and Twist Step. You will find that when you learn the Tai Chi forms, some of the movements will come to you easily and others that may look easy seem somehow elusive. Advice here is to try to understand what makes a certain movement difficult for you. If you can work this out, then you will be able to apply your knowledge to the rest of your form.

Another way of working with the same idea is to pick a movement and practise it as much as you can. If you are in a hotel room with very little space, you can normally practise one movement. As the Tai Chi sequences are designed to teach you the principles of Tai Chi through their movement, your depth of knowledge in one move-

ment can then be applied to other movements within the form.

When we practise our Tai Chi, we try as best we can to execute the movements perfectly. Even the most skilled masters still do not regard their Tai Chi as perfect. This suggests that Tai Chi is a very rich source from which we can teach ourselves something about self-improvement.

Many of the more commercially-oriented teachers will ignore this fact and try to teach their students as many different forms as possible. This denies the student the chance to study any one form in depth and real learning becomes difficult. There is a piece of Chinese wisdom that warns you that a person who knows many martial arts movements is less dangerous than a person who understands only one. There is a difference between a movement and understanding it.

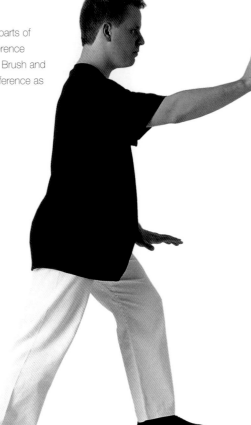

The movements of the Tai Chi form work different parts of your body in different ways. You may see little difference between White Crane Spreads its Wings (left) and Brush and Push (right) at first glance, but you will learn the difference as you study the form.

Characteristics of Tai Chi styles

We know that there are different Tai Chi styles and that the main style covered in this book is Yang style, but how does this differ from other styles? When you have more experience of watching the different Tai Chi forms, you will be able to recognise them instantly. This is not from knowing the other styles in depth, but you pick up something of their general flavour by watching them.

As a quick, and by no means definitive guide, the flavours for the Yang, Chen and Wu styles are outlined below.

Yang Style

This contains all soft movements. There is very little use of low postures but a common use of 'Ward off' energy.

An example of the Yang style, used throughout this book. All the movements are soft.

Chen style

Contains explosive fast movements as well as soft movements. There is frequent use of low postures, and it uses more elbowing techniques than the Yang style.

Wu style

Again, this contains all soft movements. It is more upright than either the Yang or the Chen styles. In general, the waist turns but the hips are stationary. There is extensive use of the space between thumb and forefinger.

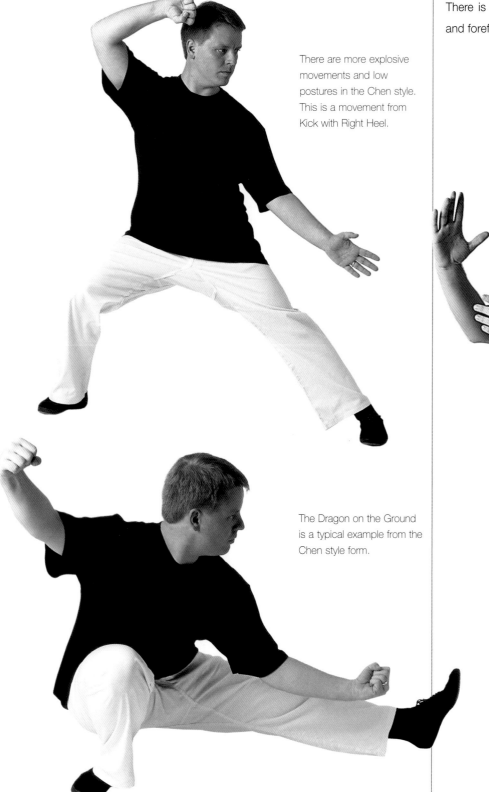

There are more explosive movements and low postures in the Chen style. This is a movement from Kick with Right Heel.

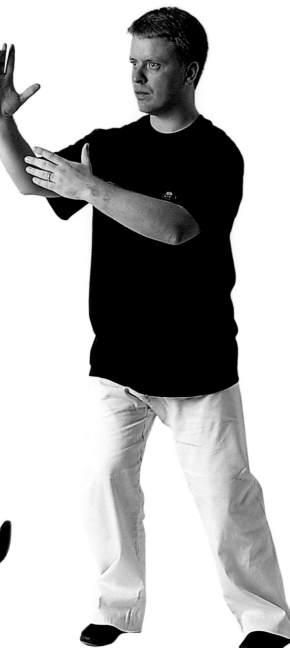

The Wu style also involves soft movements. It is an upright style, and uses the space between thumb and forefinger extensively.

The Dragon on the Ground is a typical example from the Chen style form.

LEARNING THE TAI CHI FORM

We are now ready to start learning how to do the form. The first thing that you need to understand is the use of stances. We use properly defined stances in martial arts because they are designed through the experience of the Masters to be the strongest for the particular application. Many martial art stances may look very similar, but you will find that they are subtly different. For example, the Bow Stance in Tai Chi looks similar to a karate front stance. The karate stance will normally be longer and lower than the Tai Chi stance. Remember that one is NOT better than the other; it is simply that Tai Chi uses your body in different ways.

The Stances

Apart from the Wu Chi position that we have already discussed, there are two more stances to learn.

Bow Stance is used in Parting the Wild Horse's Mane; Brush Knee and Twist Step; Grasp the Sparrow's Tail; Single Whip; Fair Lady works Shuttles; Fan through the Back; Parry, Block and Punch and Apparent Close-up.

Empty Stance is used in White Crane Spreads its Wings and Strum the Lute.

If you find that you are standing in any other stance during the form, this must be corrected. It is therefore essential to gain a thorough understanding of the postures before you start.

Bow Stance

In Bow Stance, the weight is approximately 70 per cent on the front leg and 30 per cent on the back leg. There are two variations of the Bow Stance. In one the torso of the body and the back leg are straight, and in the other the torso is vertical.

Getting into Bow Stance

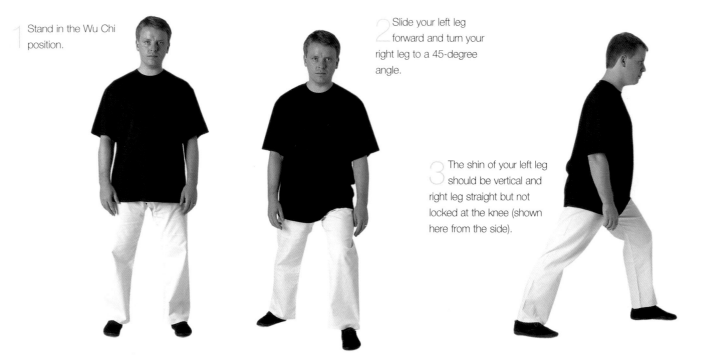

1 Stand in the Wu Chi position.

2 Slide your left leg forward and turn your right leg to a 45-degree angle.

3 The shin of your left leg should be vertical and right leg straight but not locked at the knee (shown here from the side).

Empty Stance

The empty stance is regarded by many as the most difficult. This is because all of the weight is supported on the back leg.

Getting into Empty Stance

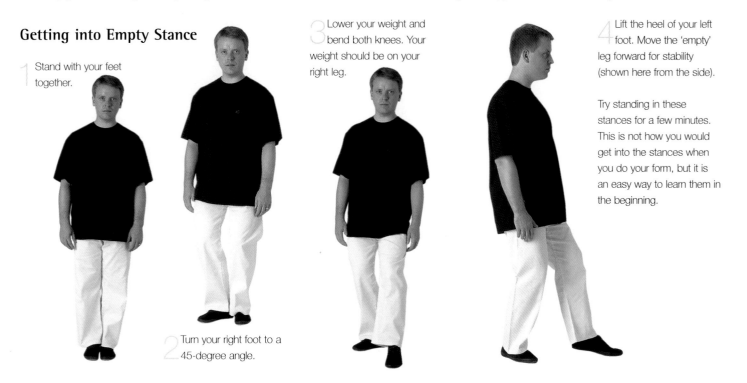

1 Stand with your feet together.

2 Turn your right foot to a 45-degree angle.

3 Lower your weight and bend both knees. Your weight should be on your right leg.

4 Lift the heel of your left foot. Move the 'empty' leg forward for stability (shown here from the side).

Try standing in these stances for a few minutes. This is not how you would get into the stances when you do your form, but it is an easy way to learn them in the beginning.

The Tai Chi walk

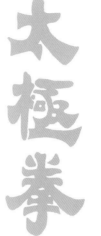

Now that you know the stances in Tai Chi, the next thing to understand is how to move in them. The most common and effective way of doing this is to learn the Tai Chi walk. Everything that you do in the Tai Chi form is deliberate and with intent. How you walk needs attention before you try to learn some of the more advanced aspects.

If you can get your stance right in Tai Chi, you are making good inroads into the form. If you practise your stances as in the last chapter, you get the basic idea, but when you step forward, the stance will become incorrect without serious training. The Tai Chi walk is an easy way to teach your legs to move into the right position. It also has the advantage of being fairly simple. When you practise the Tai Chi walk, you do not need to use your arms. This means that all of your attention will be directed to your legs and helps you to ground your energy.

Practising the Tai Chi walk

1 Stand in the Wu Chi Position.

2 Slide your right leg forward into the Bow Stance and twist your left foot to a 45-degree angle. Your weight should be 70 per cent on your right leg.

3 Sink your weight back onto your left leg. Keep your back straight and turn your waist to the right. Lift the toes of your right toe but keep the heel in contact with the floor. Your weight should be 100% on your left leg.

When you have moved on and no longer consider yourself to be a beginner, do not forget the Tai Chi walk. If you get to this stage, you will still be working on getting your stances right and the Tai Chi walk will help you jump to an intermediate level of skill.

All of the stepping movements in section one are done in the Bow Stance. The Tai Chi walk that we practise here will, therefore, be moving forward in the Bow Stance.

Once you have followed the instructions below, you will have completed one full step in the Bow Stance. Repeat the movement with the other leg. Continue the Tai Chi walk for long enough to feel the effort.

If you are doing it correctly, you will find that all of the weight changes are fairly strenuous at first, so take it easy. After practising the Tai Chi walk for a few weeks it will seem effortless. This is one of the first milestones of your Tai Chi journey.

4 Put the toe of your right foot on the floor. Push your weight from your left leg to your right leg. Keep your back straight.

5 When you have transferred ALL of your weight onto your right leg, you will be able to pick up your left leg without wobbling. Pick up the heel before the toe.

6 Step straight through with your left leg. Be aware of where you are going to put your foot so that you finish in the Bow Stance. Place the foot down with heel first and then toe.

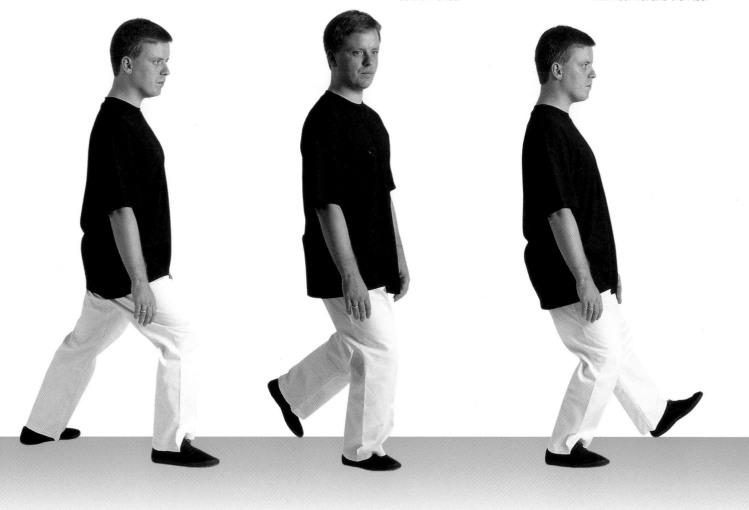

Hand positions

太極拳

Now that we have worked on the footwork, the next general set of principles belongs to the hands. There are only three actual shapes for the hands in the simplified Tai Chi form. These are the open hand, 'tigers mouth' and fist. During the form, there will be countless processes happening within the person practising. If you are trying to remember the sequence amd all you have learnt, extremities of the body such as hands and feet are easily forgotten. If you have clarity in the beginning, then you are more likely to keep them correct.

If you have managed to achieve a skill level where you do not need to try to remember the form, then you will be able to give more of your attention to your hands. When you no longer need to try to position your hands correctly, you can transfer your attention to another aspect of Tai Chi.

Too limp

Too tight

Correct position

Open hand (Tai Chi palm)

During Tai Chi practice, a common mistake is to hold your hands limp. This stops energy from travelling to your fingertips and they will appear lifeless. Limpness in the hand will also deny any understanding of martial applications, and therefore the intent will not be exercised. Without intent, you will not be able to feel the strength of the energy.

Usually after being instructed to not keep their hands limp, the student will go to the other extreme. The hand will become very tight and exert too much force. This will hinder the movement and affect the blood circulation.

The correct way of holding the hand for the Tai Chi Palm is somewhere in between the limp and the tight hand. The fingers should be extended, but they should also be relaxed. The thumb is relaxed and quite close to the hand. This allows proper circulation of blood and energy so the hands will feel more alive.

To achieve this extended but relaxed feeling with the hands, it is usual to swing between too soft and too tense in the beginning. This is a similar process to hardening and tempering a metal tool or sword. It is said that a good sword needs to be tempered many times, so do not be afraid to spend some time getting it right.

Tiger's mouth

After learning the Tai Chi palm, the 'tiger's mouth' is easy. To make the shape for tiger's mouth, simply make the Tai Chi palm and move the thumb outwards. Keep the hand relaxed but extended as before.

It is easy to slip into the tiger's mouth configuration of the hand by simply letting the thumb drift. If this happens, then you will need to pay attention to the hands, as it is incorrect.

Tiger's mouth

Tai Chi fist

Fists are used towards the latter end of the form. The fist in Tai Chi is similar to the fist used in many other martial arts, except that it is relaxed. If your fist becomes too tense, then it will be the same as having the Tai Chi palm too tense, as explained earlier.

To make the Tai Chi fist, start by making the Tai Chi palm. Now roll your fingers towards your hand, so that they touch the palm. Finish the fist by bringing your thumb down over the first two fingers.

A common mistake is to bend your wrist when making a fist. The energy to your fist should come in a straight line from your elbow. If you bend your wrist, you will simply not be able to transmit power through your fist. If you were to hit anything with a fist that was bent, you would hurt your wrist.

Tai Chi fist

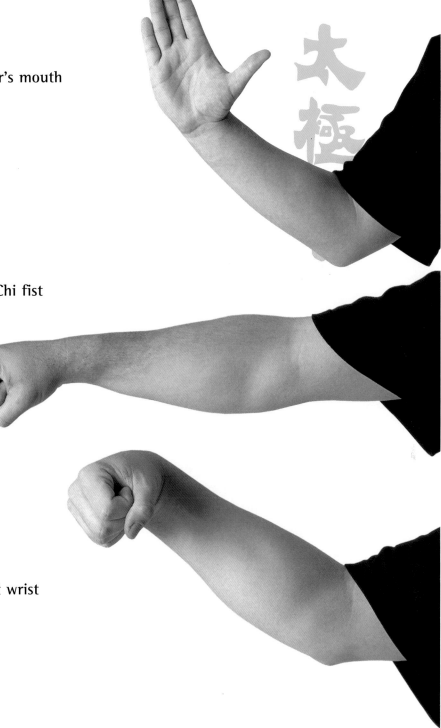

Bent wrist

Hollow fist

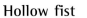

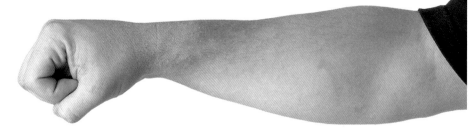

Another common mistake is to make a 'hollow' fist. This is again incorrect for the style of Tai Chi studied here.

YANG STYLE TAI CHI FORM PART ONE

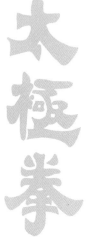

There are three sections to the Yang style Tai Chi Form. This book looks only at the first section, but examines it in depth to provide you with a greater understanding of the meaning and applications of the movements described. It is better to gain a full understanding of one part of the form, rather than a more sketchy understanding of the full form. If you wish to take your studies further, look around for a local school or instructor. You may also wish to look at different versions of the Yang style Tai Chi form – and there are many. Once you have whetted your appetite, there are a wide variety of options for you to pursue. The Yang style demonstrated here was taught to me by Shelagh Grandpierre of the Tai Chi Alliance and Master Christopher Pei of the United States Wushu Academy.

Movements of the form

The first part of the Yang style form consists of 16 movements, including some repetition. The movements are:

Opening form
Ward-off Left
Grasping the Sparrow' s Tail
Single Whip
Raise Hands
White Crane Spreads its Wings
Brush and Push 1
Strum the Lute 1
Brush and Push 2
Brush and Push 3
Brush and Push 4
Strum the Lute 2
Brush and Push 5
Parry, Block and Punch
Apparent Close-up
Cross Hands
Closing Form

For the purpose of making the form as easy to follow as possible, some of the movements have been photographed from a different angle. Where you should be facing a certain direction, this is indicated in the text.

Begin in the Wu Chi position, explained earlier in the book.

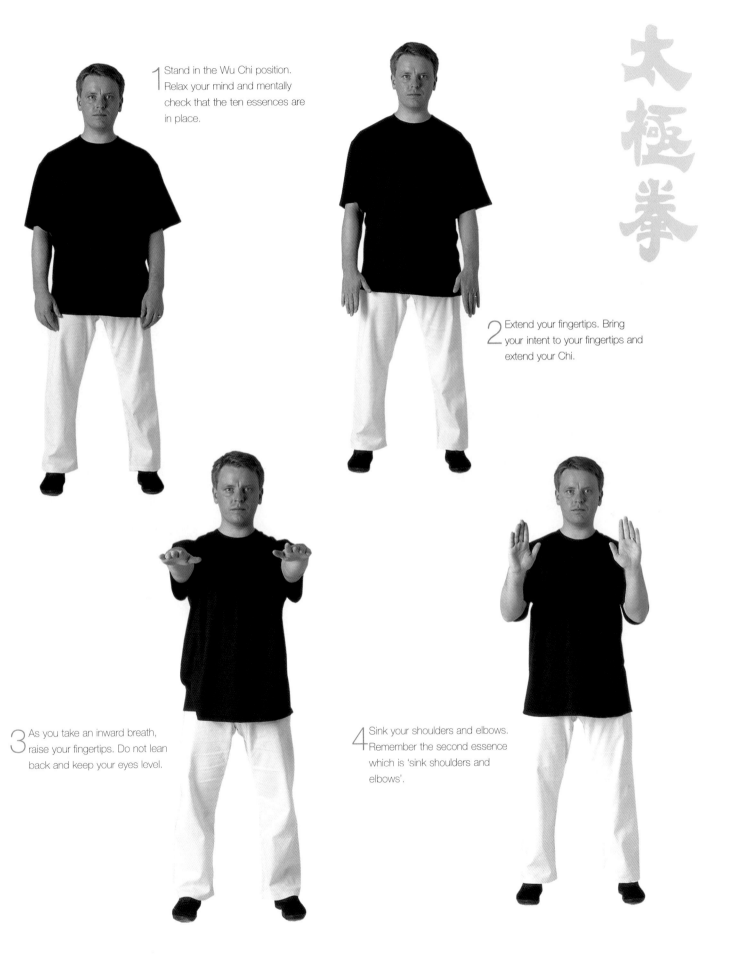

太極拳

1 Stand in the Wu Chi position. Relax your mind and mentally check that the ten essences are in place.

2 Extend your fingertips. Bring your intent to your fingertips and extend your Chi.

3 As you take an inward breath, raise your fingertips. Do not lean back and keep your eyes level.

4 Sink your shoulders and elbows. Remember the second essence which is 'sink shoulders and elbows'.

太極拳

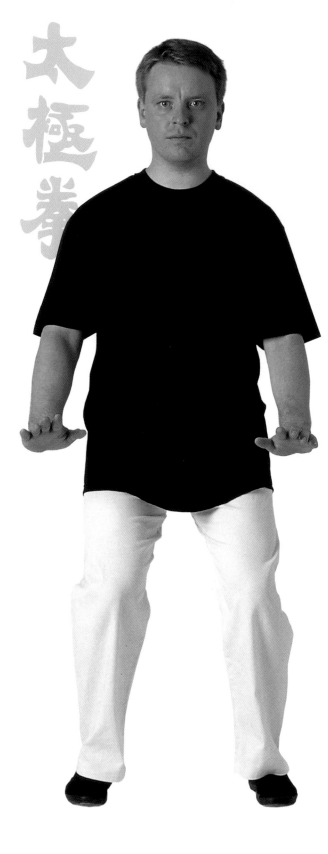

5 Press the palms of both hands to the floor. Bend your knees, as your forearms pass the Tan Tien point.

Ward-off Left

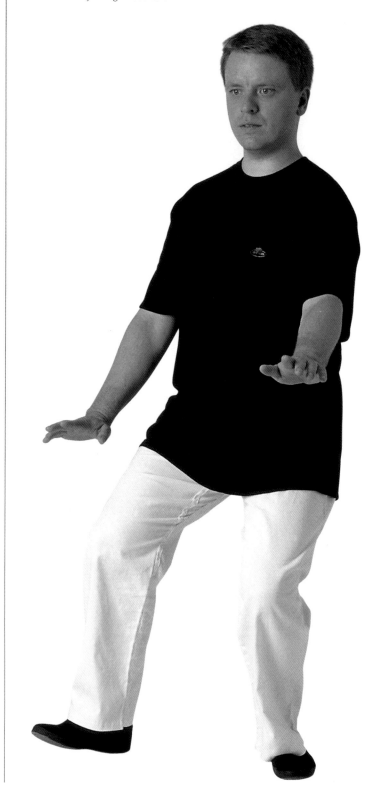

1 Rotate your waist clockwise. Pull your right hand back and push your left hand forward. Shift your weight onto your right leg. Turn the toes of your right foot 45°.

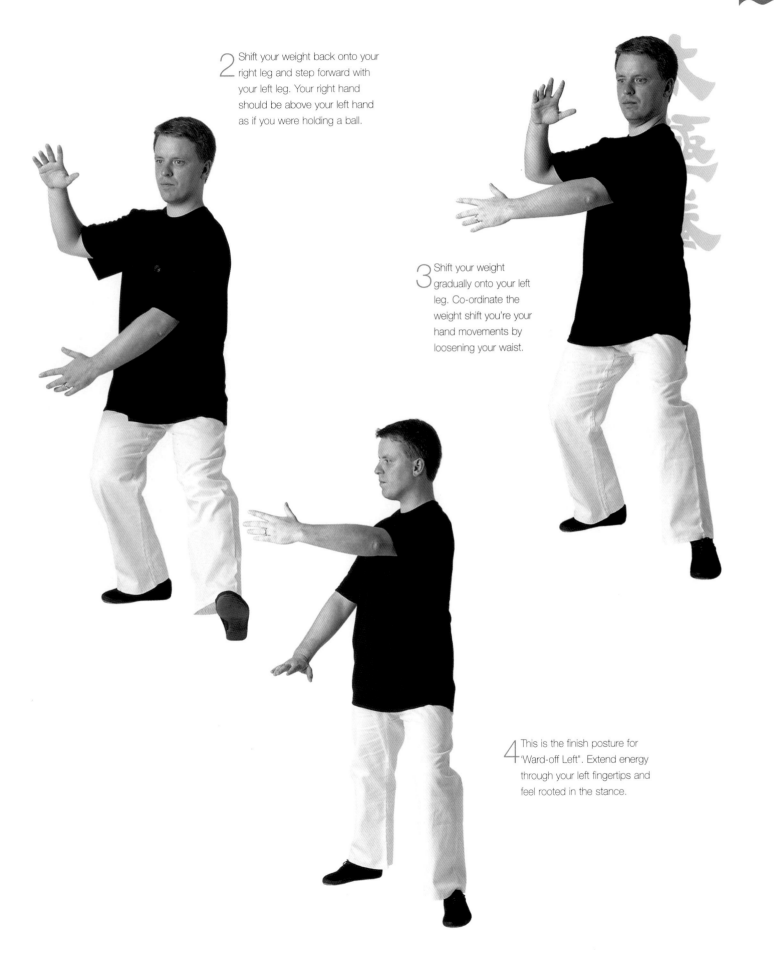

2 Shift your weight back onto your right leg and step forward with your left leg. Your right hand should be above your left hand as if you were holding a ball.

3 Shift your weight gradually onto your left leg. Co-ordinate the weight shift you're your hand movements by loosening your waist.

4 This is the finish posture for 'Ward-off Left'. Extend energy through your left fingertips and feel rooted in the stance.

Grasping the Sparrow's Tail

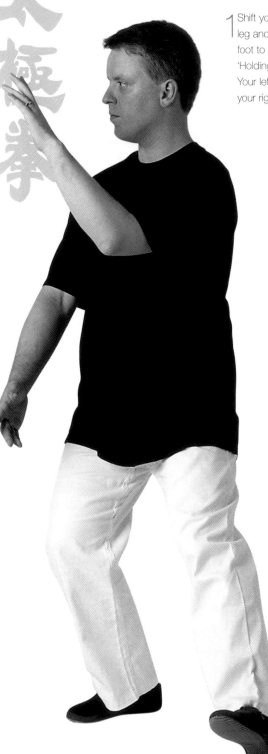

1 Shift your weight onto your right leg and turn the toes of your left foot to a 45° angle. Make the 'Holding Ball' form with your arms. Your left arm should be above your right arm.

2 Shift your weight over to your left leg. There should be no weight in your right leg. Simply relax your shoulders and elbows.

3 Step forward with your right leg. Do not transfer weight yet. Your step should come down heel first, followed by the ball of your foot.

4 Ward-off on Right Side. Push your weight from your left leg to your right. This finishes the 'Ward-off Right Side' part of the sequence. Remember to keep a good Bow Stance.

5 Rotate your waist in a clockwise direction. Extend your arms and keep your elbow joints soft.

6 Rotate your waist anti-clockwise and start to shift your weight back onto your left leg.

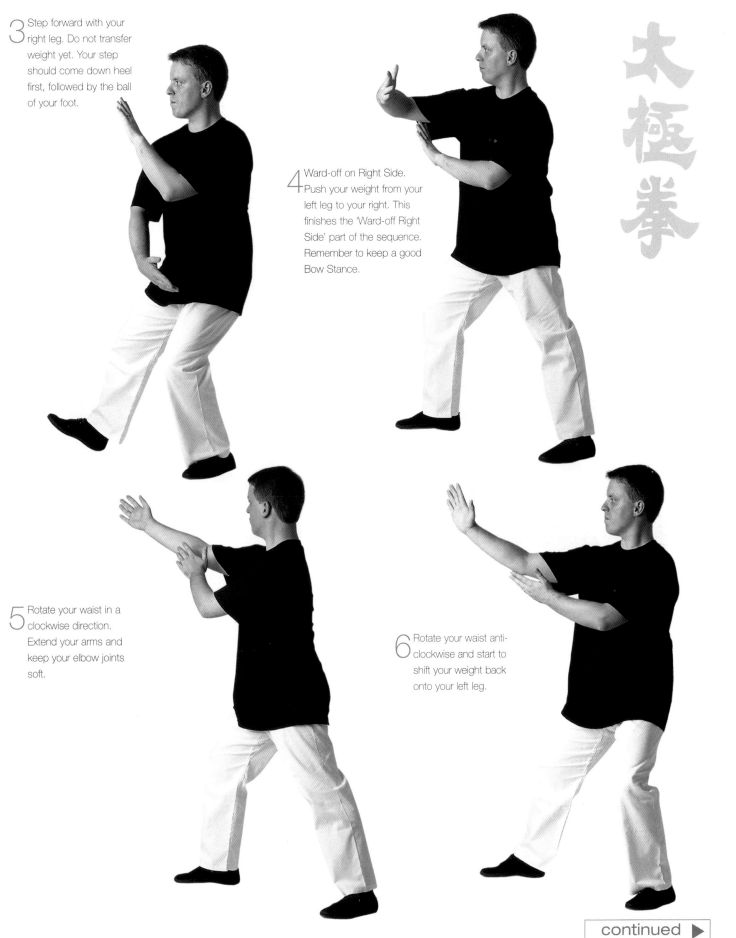

continued ▶

Grasping the Sparrow's Tail continued

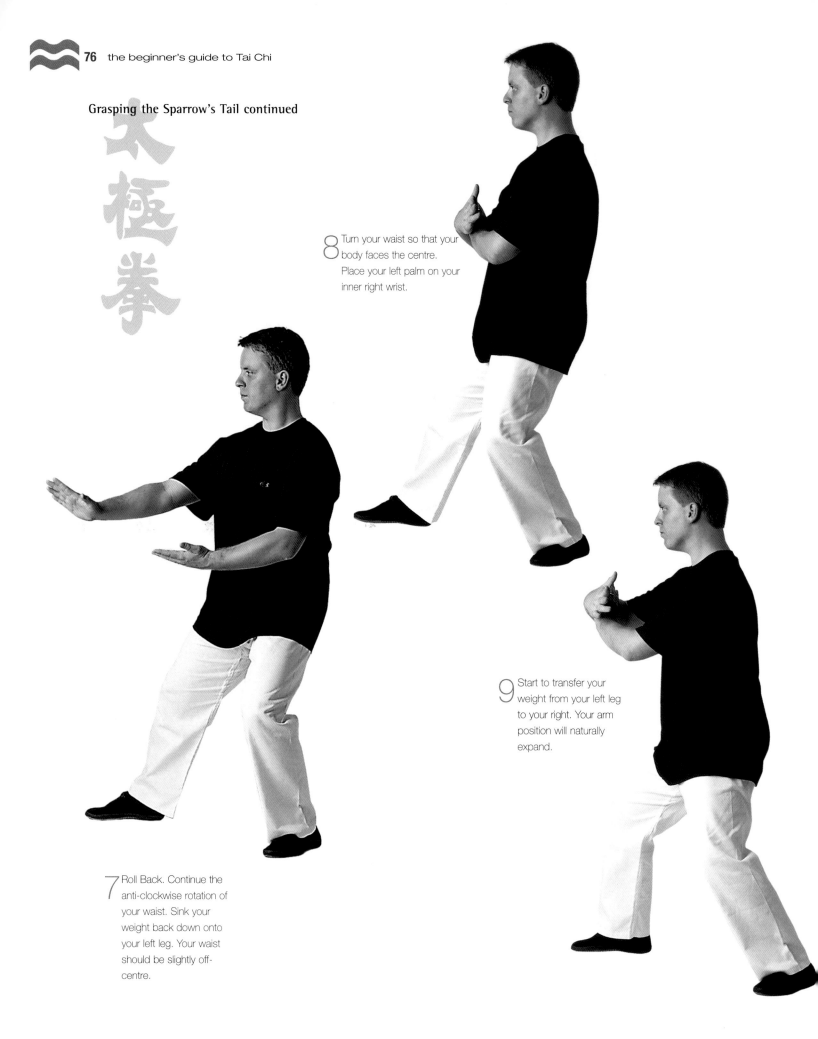

8 Turn your waist so that your body faces the centre. Place your left palm on your inner right wrist.

9 Start to transfer your weight from your left leg to your right. Your arm position will naturally expand.

7 Roll Back. Continue the anti-clockwise rotation of your waist. Sink your weight back down onto your left leg. Your waist should be slightly off-centre.

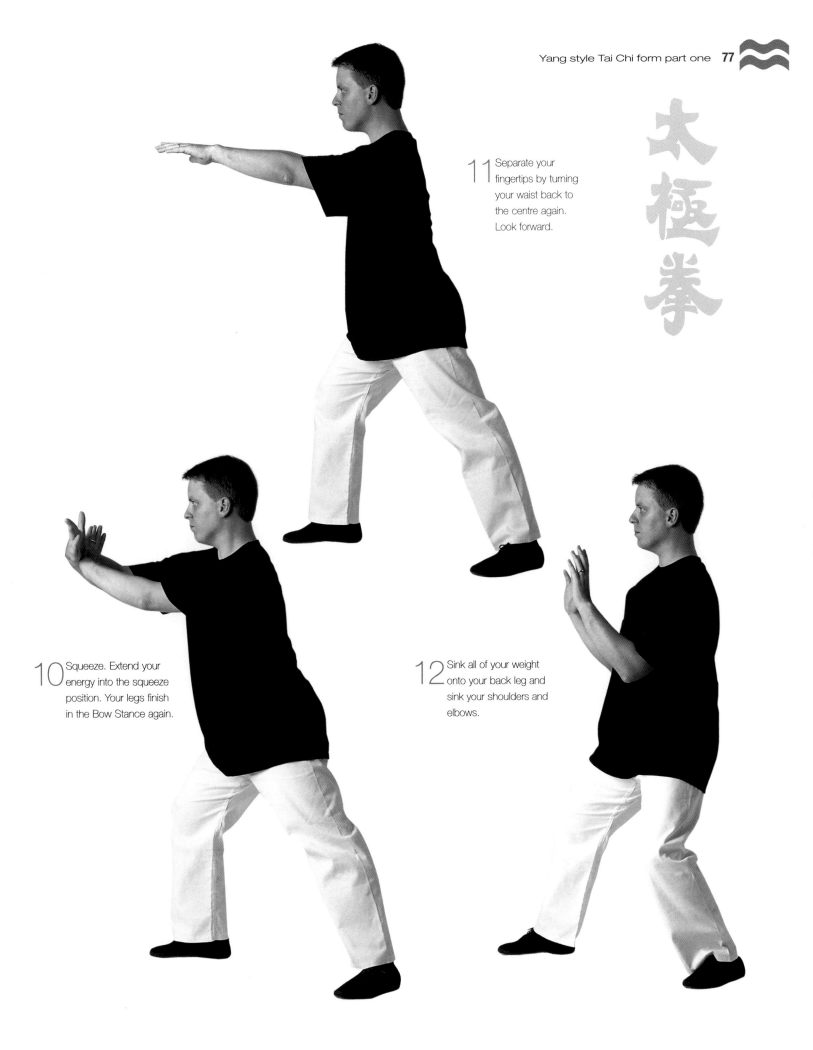

太極拳

11 Separate your fingertips by turning your waist back to the centre again. Look forward.

10 Squeeze. Extend your energy into the squeeze position. Your legs finish in the Bow Stance again.

12 Sink all of your weight onto your back leg and sink your shoulders and elbows.

Grasping the Sparrow's Tail continued

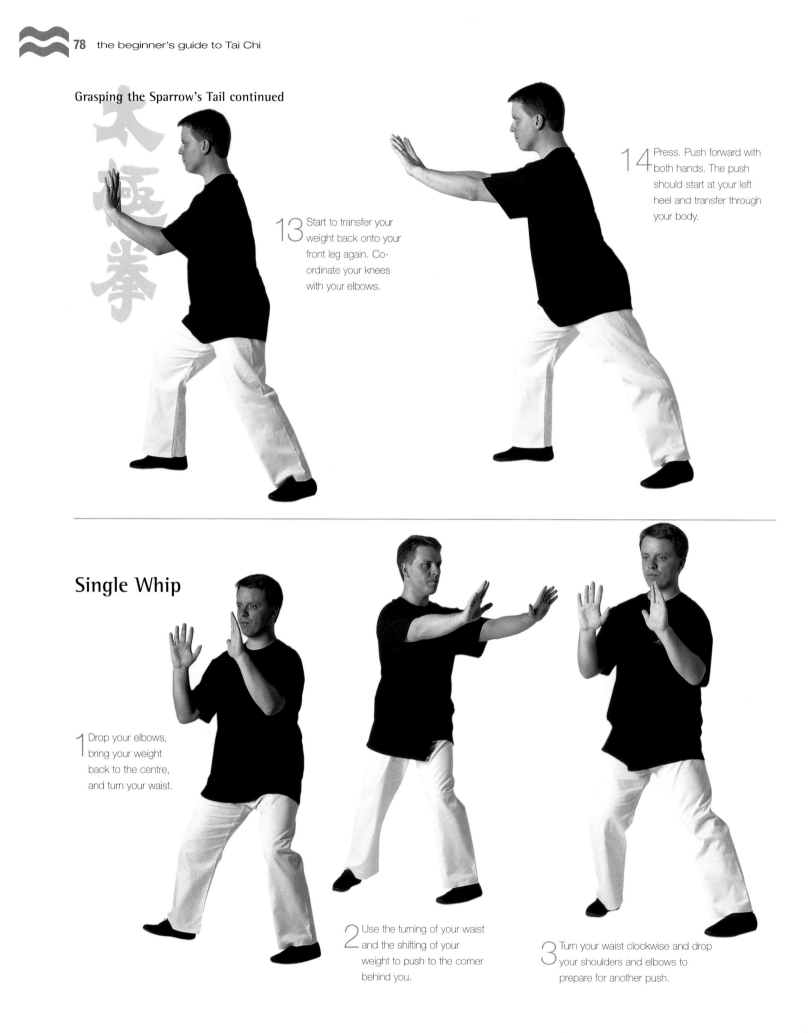

13 Start to transfer your weight back onto your front leg again. Co-ordinate your knees with your elbows.

14 Press. Push forward with both hands. The push should start at your left heel and transfer through your body.

Single Whip

1 Drop your elbows, bring your weight back to the centre, and turn your waist.

2 Use the turning of your waist and the shifting of your weight to push to the corner behind you.

3 Turn your waist clockwise and drop your shoulders and elbows to prepare for another push.

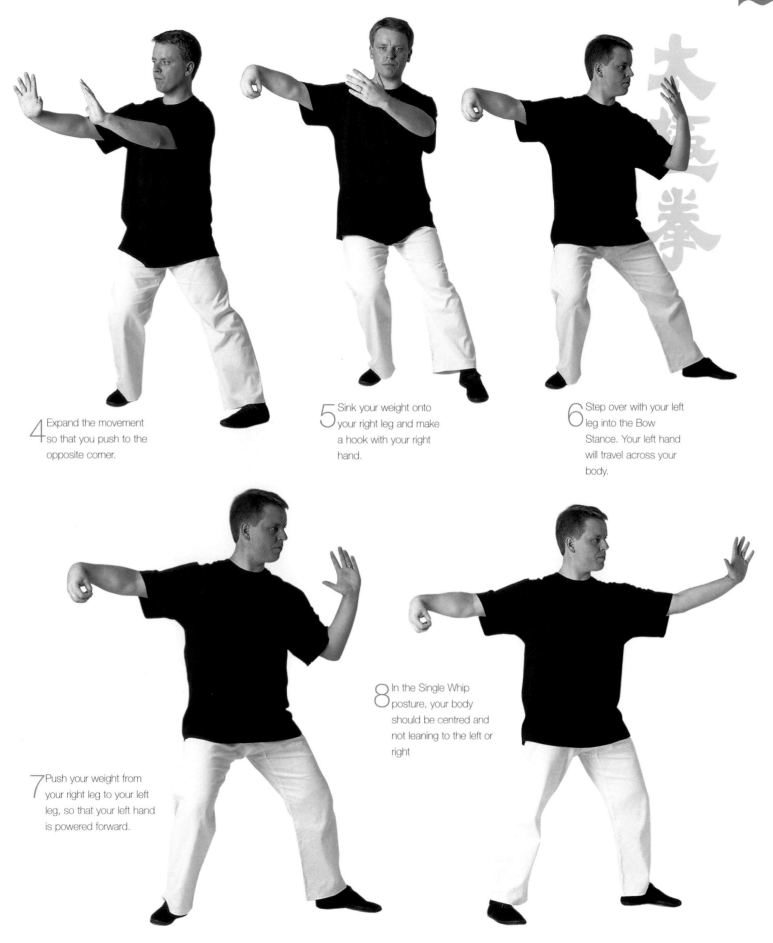

4 Expand the movement so that you push to the opposite corner.

5 Sink your weight onto your right leg and make a hook with your right hand.

6 Step over with your left leg into the Bow Stance. Your left hand will travel across your body.

7 Push your weight from your right leg to your left leg, so that your left hand is powered forward.

8 In the Single Whip posture, your body should be centred and not leaning to the left or right

Raise Hands

1 Press all of your weight down onto your right leg, and turn your left foot 45°. Open your hands.

2 Shift your weight onto your left leg as you turn your waist and close your hands.

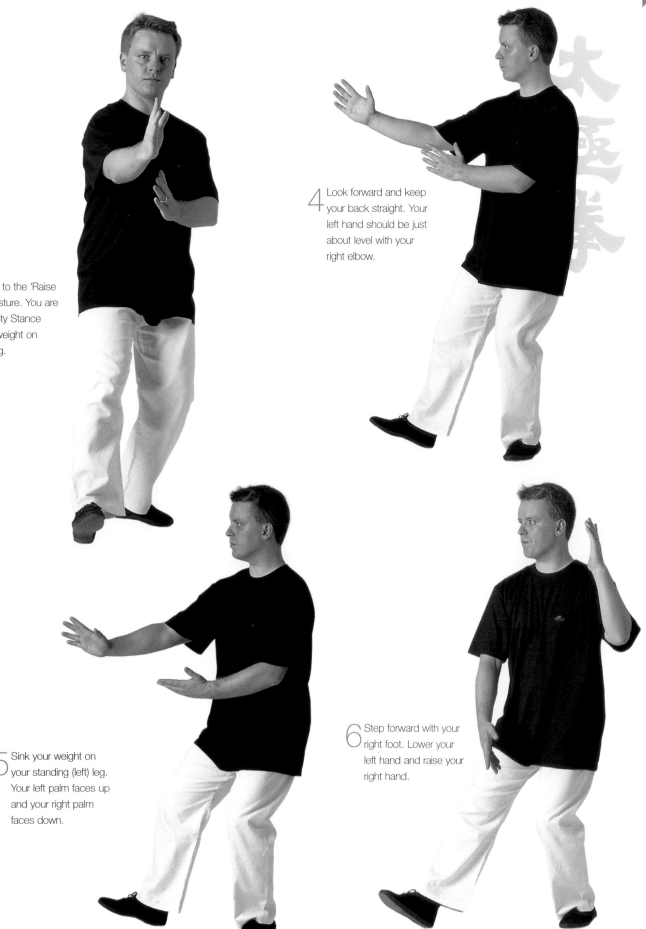

3 Sink down to the 'Raise Hands' posture. You are in the Empty Stance with your weight on your left leg.

4 Look forward and keep your back straight. Your left hand should be just about level with your right elbow.

5 Sink your weight on your standing (left) leg. Your left palm faces up and your right palm faces down.

6 Step forward with your right foot. Lower your left hand and raise your right hand.

Raise Hands continued

太極拳

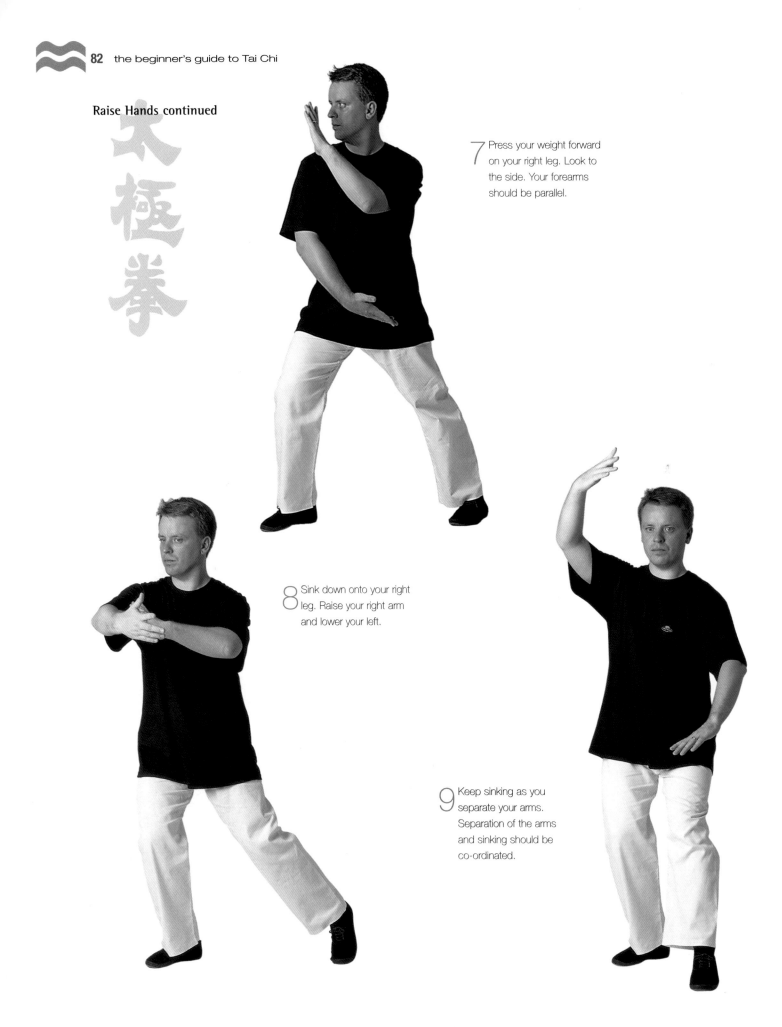

7 Press your weight forward on your right leg. Look to the side. Your forearms should be parallel.

8 Sink down onto your right leg. Raise your right arm and lower your left.

9 Keep sinking as you separate your arms. Separation of the arms and sinking should be co-ordinated.

White Crane Spreads its Wings

1 Sink into the Empty Stance. Press down with your left hand and up with your right.

2 This side view clearly shows that your back should be straight and your weight settled onto your right leg.

3 Lower your right forearm with the palm facing up. Generate power by sinking.

4 Pull your right elbow back and sweep your left arm in front of your body.

5 Step forward with your left leg. Press down with your right palm and bring your right hand back.

Brush and Push 1

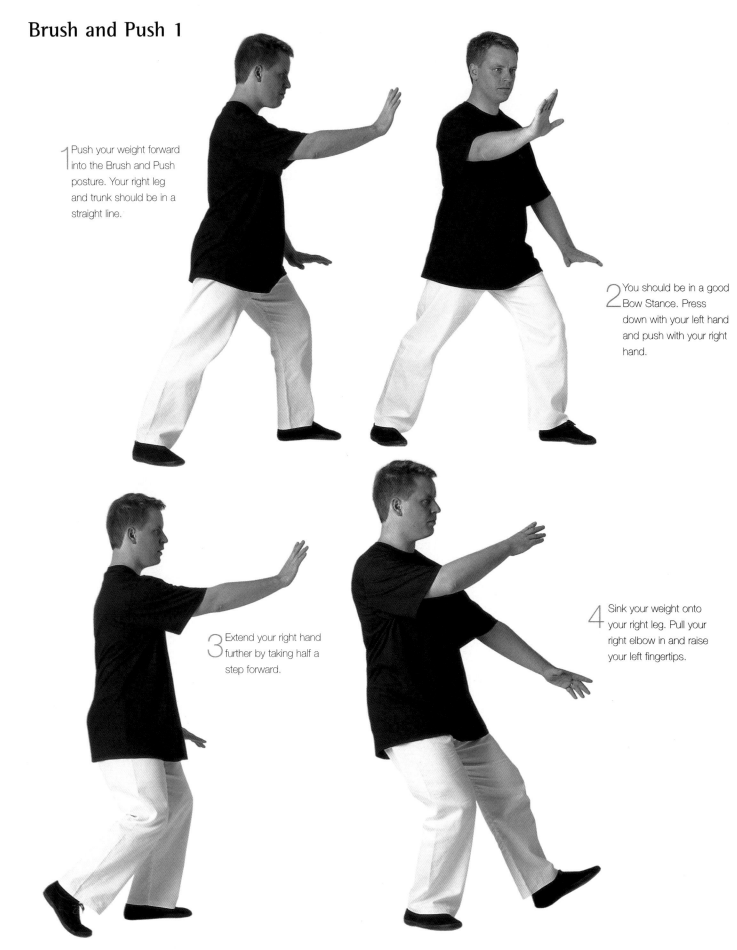

1 Push your weight forward into the Brush and Push posture. Your right leg and trunk should be in a straight line.

2 You should be in a good Bow Stance. Press down with your left hand and push with your right hand.

3 Extend your right hand further by taking half a step forward.

4 Sink your weight onto your right leg. Pull your right elbow in and raise your left fingertips.

Strum the Lute 1

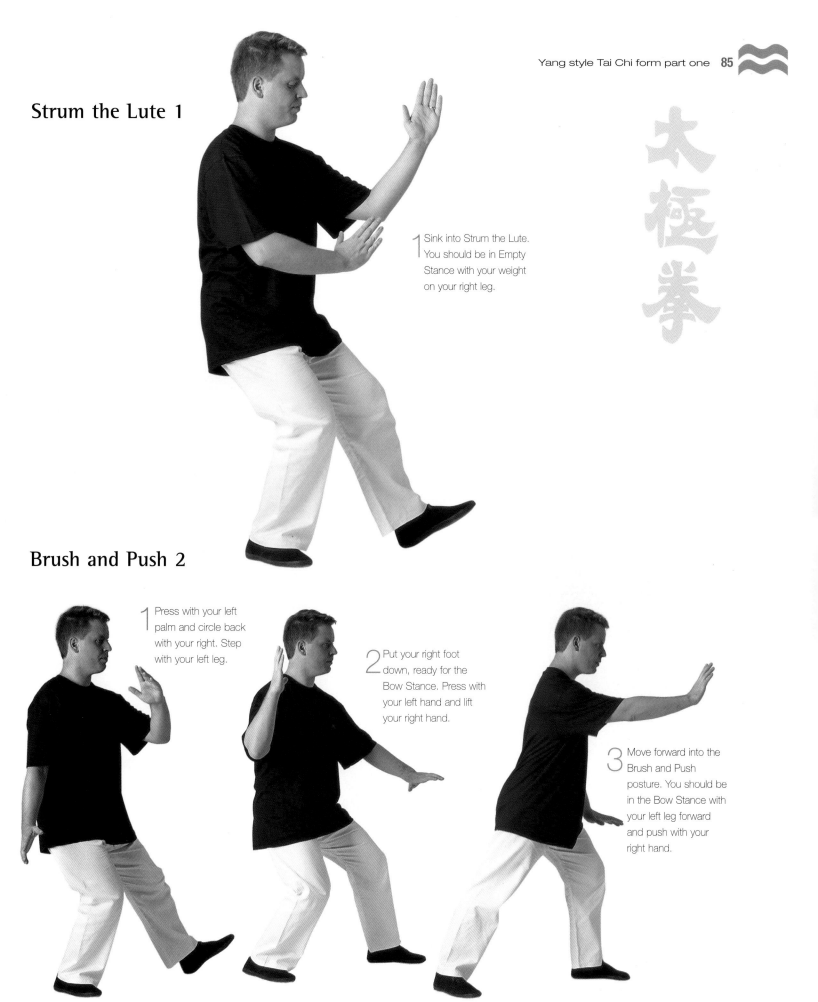

1 Sink into Strum the Lute. You should be in Empty Stance with your weight on your right leg.

Brush and Push 2

1 Press with your left palm and circle back with your right. Step with your left leg.

2 Put your right foot down, ready for the Bow Stance. Press with your left hand and lift your right hand.

3 Move forward into the Brush and Push posture. You should be in the Bow Stance with your left leg forward and push with your right hand.

Brush and Push 3

太極拳

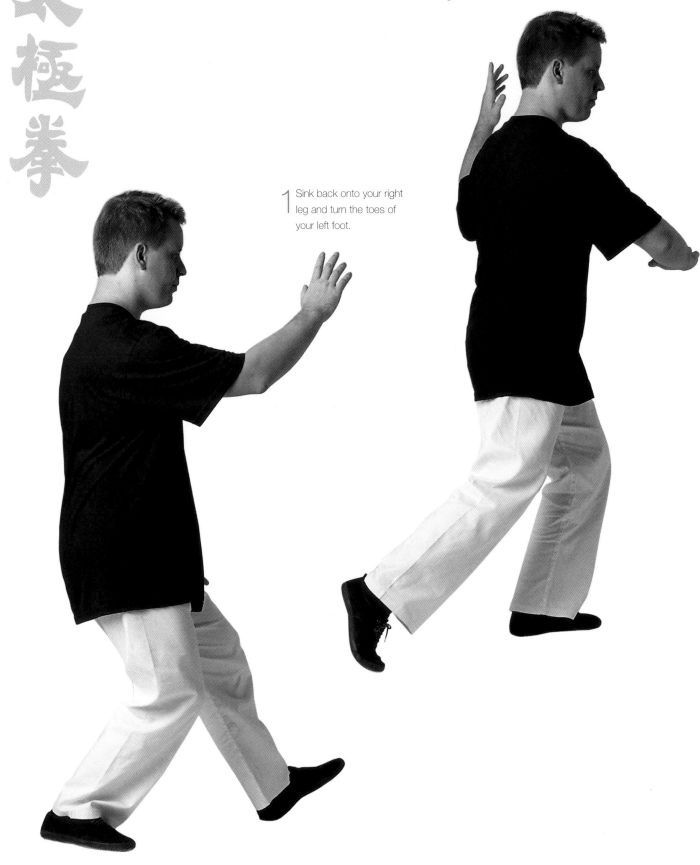

1 Sink back onto your right leg and turn the toes of your left foot.

2 Shift your weight onto your left foot and lift your right heel.

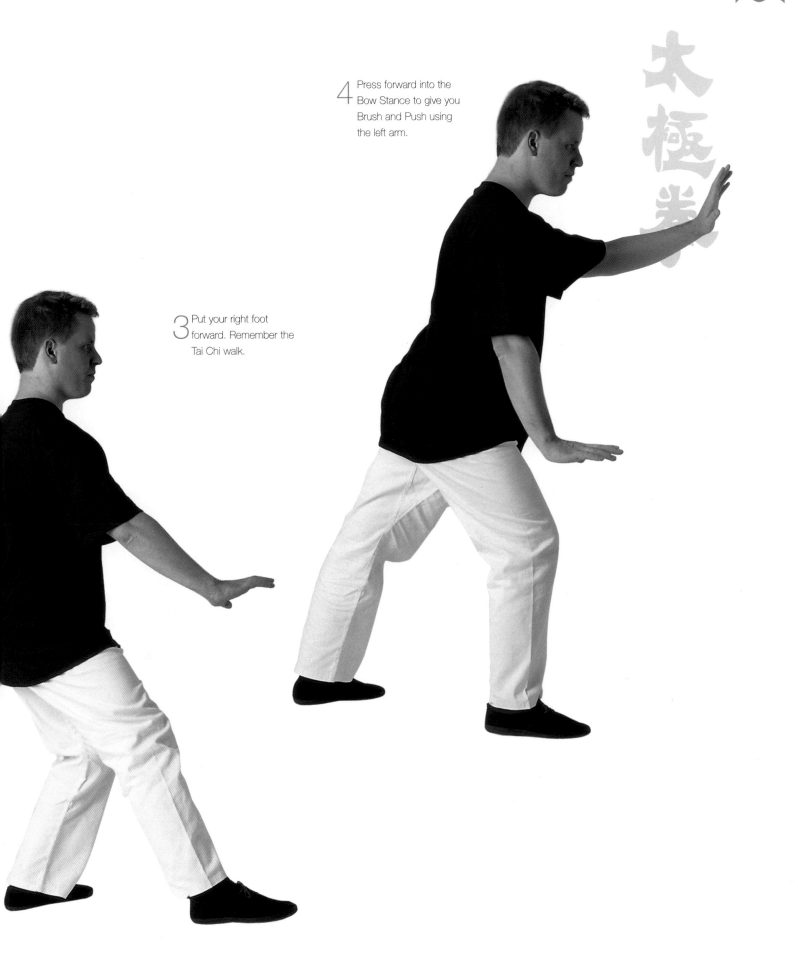

4 Press forward into the Bow Stance to give you Brush and Push using the left arm.

3 Put your right foot forward. Remember the Tai Chi walk.

Brush and Push 4

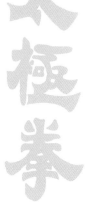

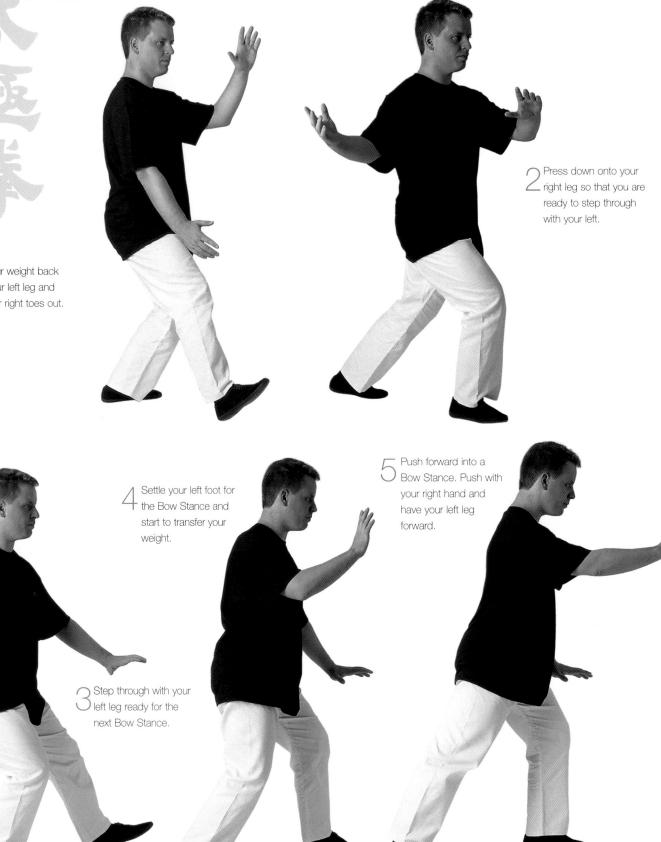

1 Sink your weight back onto your left leg and turn your right toes out.

2 Press down onto your right leg so that you are ready to step through with your left.

3 Step through with your left leg ready for the next Bow Stance.

4 Settle your left foot for the Bow Stance and start to transfer your weight.

5 Push forward into a Bow Stance. Push with your right hand and have your left leg forward.

Strum the Lute 2

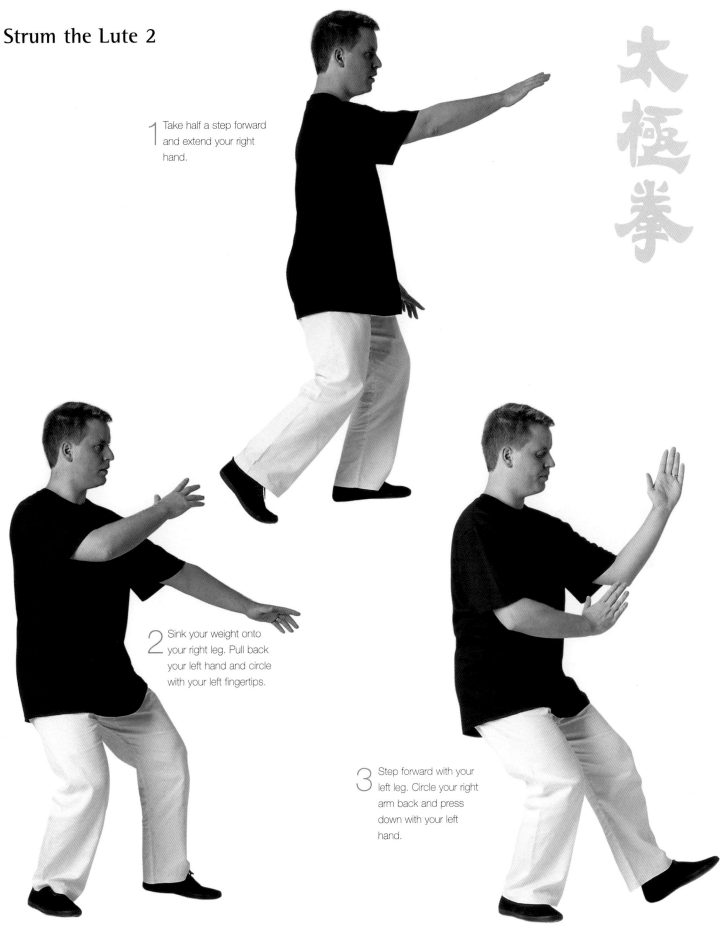

1 Take half a step forward and extend your right hand.

2 Sink your weight onto your right leg. Pull back your left hand and circle with your left fingertips.

3 Step forward with your left leg. Circle your right arm back and press down with your left hand.

Brush and Push 5

太極拳

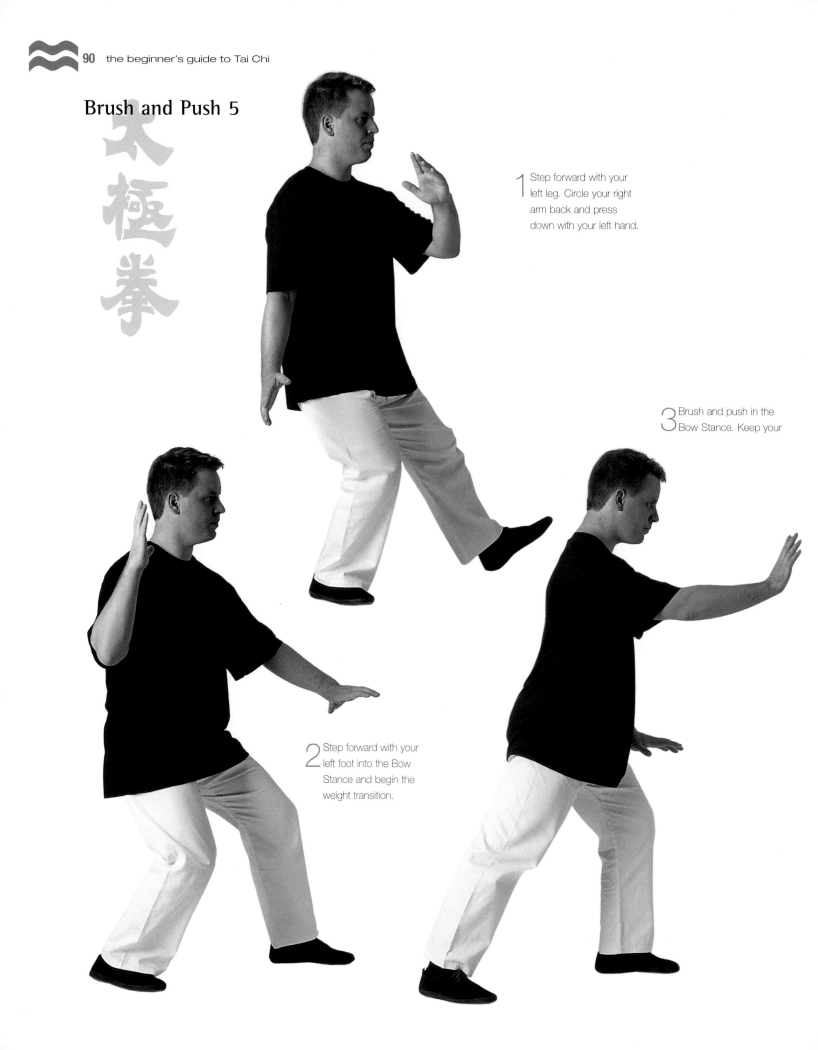

1 Step forward with your left leg. Circle your right arm back and press down with your left hand.

3 Brush and push in the Bow Stance. Keep your

2 Step forward with your left foot into the Bow Stance and begin the weight transition.

Parry, Block and Punch

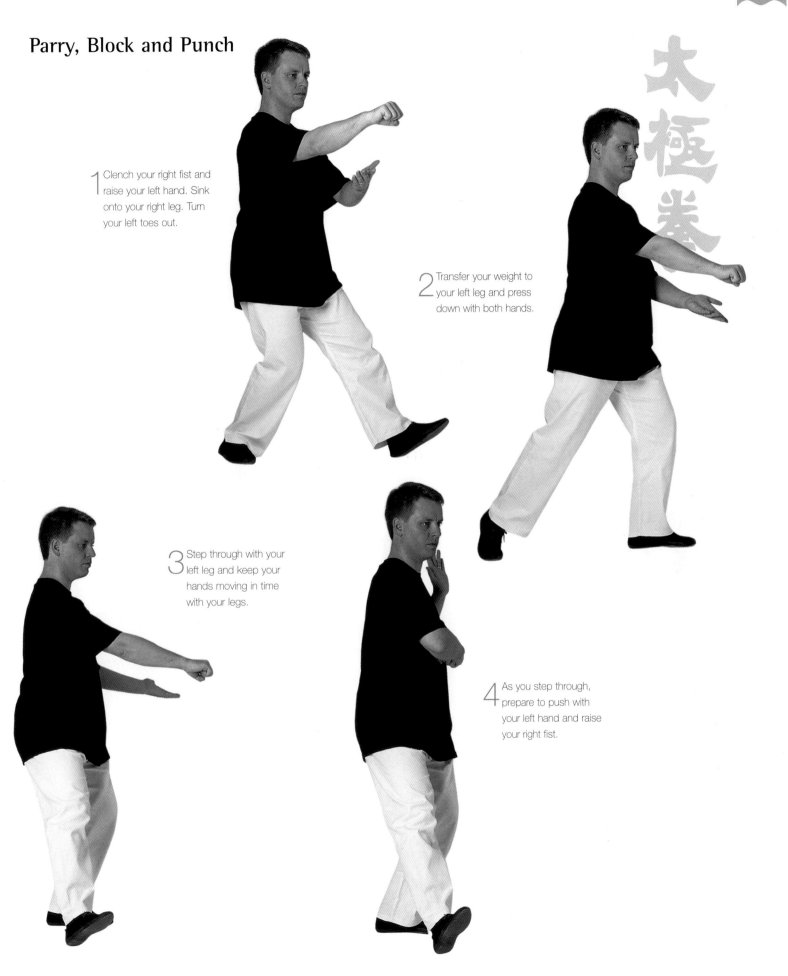

1 Clench your right fist and raise your left hand. Sink onto your right leg. Turn your left toes out.

2 Transfer your weight to your left leg and press down with both hands.

3 Step through with your left leg and keep your hands moving in time with your legs.

4 As you step through, prepare to push with your left hand and raise your right fist.

Parry, Block and Punch continued

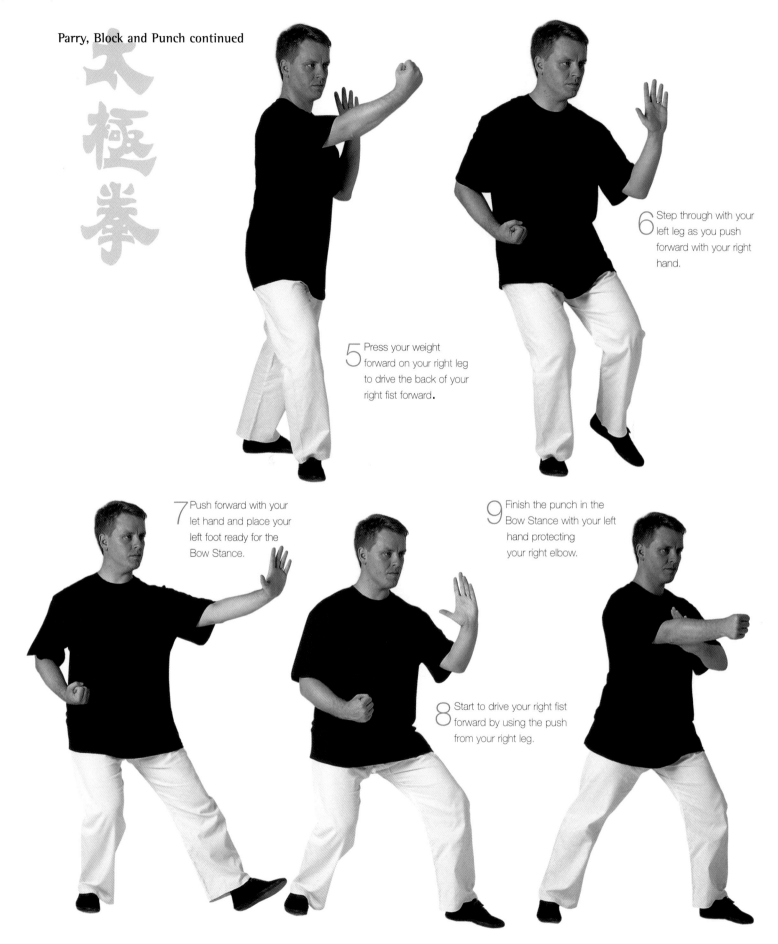

5 Press your weight forward on your right leg to drive the back of your right fist forward.

6 Step through with your left leg as you push forward with your right hand.

7 Push forward with your let hand and place your left foot ready for the Bow Stance.

8 Start to drive your right fist forward by using the push from your right leg.

9 Finish the punch in the Bow Stance with your left hand protecting your right elbow.

Apparent Close-up

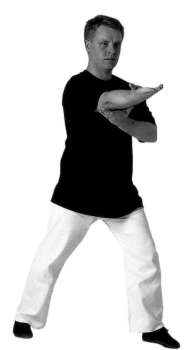

1 Open your fist and turn your hand so that the palm faces upward. Put your left hand under your right elbow.

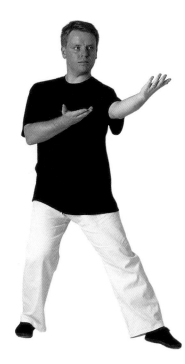

2 Twist your waist so that you pull your right hand back and push your left hand forward.

3 Sink back and drop both elbows so that you are ready to push.

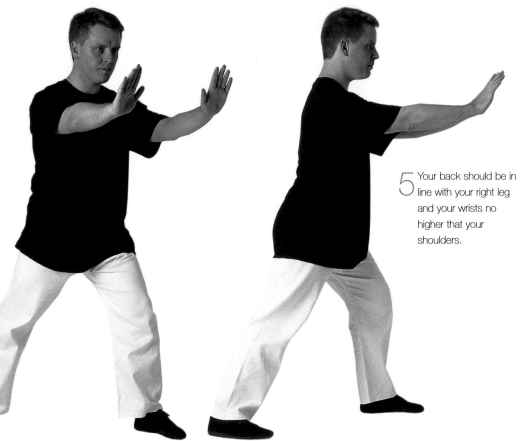

4 Push with both hands. The push should start at your right heel and travel through your body.

5 Your back should be in line with your right leg and your wrists no higher that your shoulders.

Cross Hands

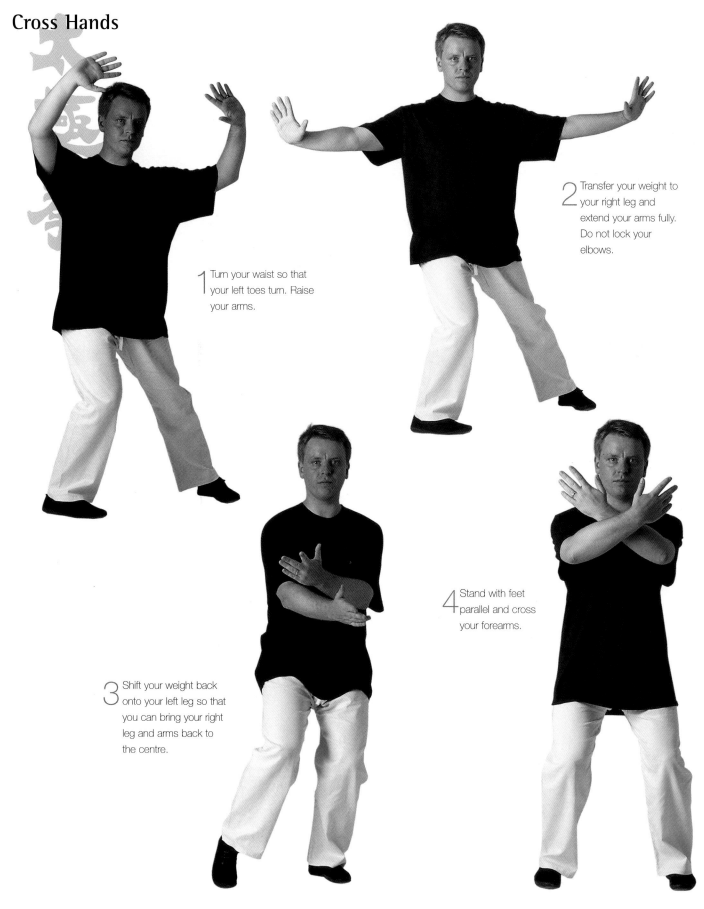

1 Turn your waist so that your left toes turn. Raise your arms.

2 Transfer your weight to your right leg and extend your arms fully. Do not lock your elbows.

3 Shift your weight back onto your left leg so that you can bring your right leg and arms back to the centre.

4 Stand with feet parallel and cross your forearms.

Closing Form

1 Open your hands and keep the palms facing upward. Keep your eyes steady and your head up.

2 Turn your arms so that your palms face the floor. Try not to lift your shoulders.

3 Lower your shoulders. Elbows, forearms and then your hands press down to the floor.

4 You have now finished section one of the form. Stand still for a short time and try to notice any internal differences.

TAI CHI POSTURE

太極拳

In Tai Chi, it is impossible to make any real progress unless you have a good understanding of posture. The mechanics of the stances and postures have been carefully improved over many years so that you can be strong within the posture. Normally if there is a physical rule such as this, it will follow with the energy in the posture. The postures are designed to open your energy meridians and teach you how to move the energy within the meridians.

How then do we learn correct posture? The first thing to remember is to take things slowly. This type of training can take lots of practise to perfect. During your practice, you need to know that you are practising the right way. It is true that practice makes perfect, but you have to get your practising right. If you continually practise the wrong way, then you will waste time. To ensure that your practice is correct, you need a good teacher. It also helps if you understand what you are doing. When you are trying to understand your Tai Chi movements, the Ten Essences are your most powerful tools. If you are doing something that does not satisfy the conditions of the Ten Essences, you are doing something wrong.

Posture in Tai Chi is not just about the physical alignment of your body. Take the first Essence, 'lift the head to raise the spirit'. If you understand this Essence, you will always know where to look. If your eyes are on your feet all the time, how can you raise your spirit? This observation alone is enough to give you the edge over many other Tai Chi students (and some masters!)

In Tai Chi you should always be looking ahead. This will keep your spirit and strength high.

If you are constantly looking at your hands, your will look defeated before you begin!

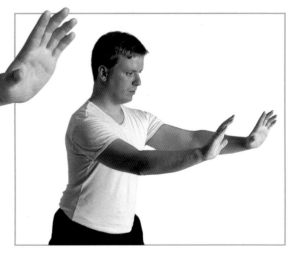

Body alignment

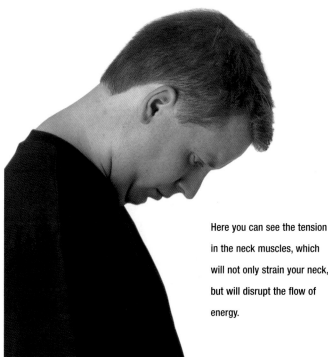

Here you can see the tension in the neck muscles, which will not only strain your neck, but will disrupt the flow of energy.

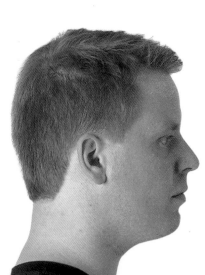

Correct posture involves keeping muscles relaxed, aiding energy flow and prevention pain and strain.

Tai Chi theory agrees with other methods such as the Alexander Technique in that it is of primary importance to gain an understanding of the relationship between your neck, head and back.

The head is a fairly heavy weight, with the average being approximately 3.5 kg (7$^3/_4$ lb). Its centre of gravity is slightly forward of the mid line. This is demonstrated by the fact that you tilt your head forward if you fall asleep in a sitting position.

If your head is in a tilted position, it will put strain on your vertebrae and spine. This can cause structural damage to your neck. Just think about how many people get stiff necks, etc.

If you consider that your body can be regarded mechanically as a series of objects in a stack, then you cannot achieve good balance unless the heavy object at the top is balanced.

This balancing is not something that can be achieved overnight. If you have a habitual pattern of leaning forward with your neck, it will take practise and patience to get out of that habit. Breaking any habit can be difficult enough and this is probably one that you have been unconsciously doing for years.

The muscles at the back of the neck are important considerations here. If they are not relaxed and toned, you may have a tendency towards bad neck position. This can also be exaggerated by sitting or standing in bad posture for hours at works.

How do we improve this aspect? The first thing is to be aware of your position. If you are sitting at your computer, keep checking whether or not you are stooping. Adjust your position regularly and move about as frequently as you can to loosen your body.

Another way of improving is through practising the Tai Chi form and associated exercises. This will help you to line your body into better posture and loosen your muscles.

Remember again the first Essence 'lift the head to raise the spirit'. The above considerations are all connected to that Essence. It is impossible to sink your shoulders, as in the second Essence without keeping your head up.

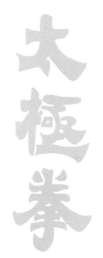

Remember the first Essence – lift your head to raise your spirit.

Standing exercises

The following exercises will teach you how to adjust your position and how to help others adjust theirs. Remember that by helping others to understand, you will also improve your own understanding.

Getting it wrong

If you can feel what happens to your body when it is incorrectly aligned, you will understand why you should try for better alignment.

1 Stand in any position – this part of the exercise needs you to be standing incorrectly.

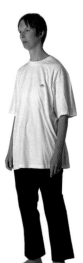

2 Your training partner should place their hands on your shoulders and press down. After very little pressure, you will feel something give way and your posture will collapse.

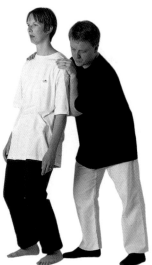

Getting it right

1 Stand in the Wu Chi position. Mentally relax your body from the top downwards. You may need your training partner to help you. Start from the crown of your head; work through your neck and shoulders and all the way down to your ankles and feet. Your partner should GRADUALLY apply pressure to your shoulders. As the pressure begins to build up, the weakest part of your posture will start to fail first. If, for instance, it is your lower back, you will feel a build-up of pressure in your lower back. When you feel this build up, tell your partner to stop.

2 Adjust your position with the information from last time and make improvements in the relevant areas. Ask your partner to put the pressure on again when you are ready. If you have adjusted correctly, then another part of your body will feel the pressure first. Now repeat the adjustment as before. When you have achieved the correct alignment, all of your training partner's efforts will go straight through you and be grounded into the floor.

This is a valuable exercise, as it can help you to find weak spots where you may need more work. The same sort of logic is then applied to the stances and positions in the form.

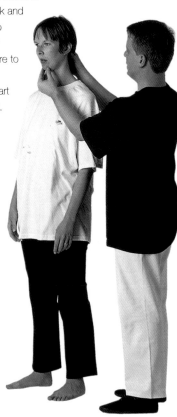

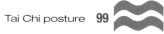

Bow Stance

Important considerations for the Bow Stance are the size of the stance itself and the position of your knee relative to your foot.

We are assuming here that you already know how to get into the Bow Stance, as described earlier.

Side Push

First, we need to check the width of the stance. The following exercises will help you with this.

1 Assume a Bow Stance, but make it too narrow (i.e. both feet nearly in line with each other).

2 Your training partner should gently push your shoulder from the side. It will take your partner very little effort to make you over-balance. They may even be able to do this with fingertip pressure.

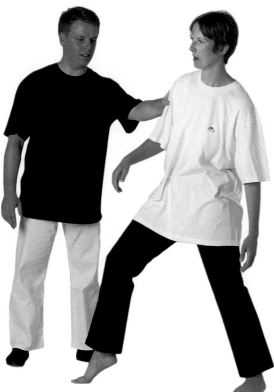

3 Bring your stance to the correct shoulder-width apart position. Your partner may help you to check your alignment if you are unsure. If your partner repeats the push to your shoulder, it will be easier for you to resist. You may find that they can still push you, but it should be much more difficult.

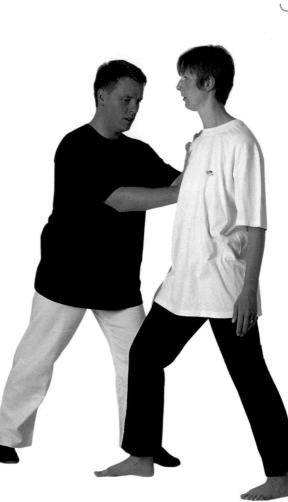

It would be logical here to suggest that a wider stance is a stronger stance. The statement has truth behind it and is exploited by some other styles. In Tai Chi, we need to be able to move in a certain way. Try to do the Tai Chi walk with a very wide stance. You will find it almost impossible to keep your balance if your stance is too wide in this exercise. The width of the stance, then, is a compromise between rigidity and movement. Ideas such as this should automatically remind you of Yin and Yang

Front Push

The real strength of the Bow Stance lies in the power of its forward Energy. This is tested as follows.

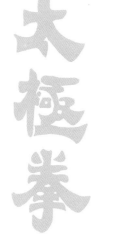

2 Your training partner should then push on your shoulders. At the weak part of your stance, you will start to buckle, so stop.

1 Assume a Bow Stance. Do not pay any particular attention to detail. Cross your arms in front of you.

3 Now adjust the Bow Stance to be as correct as you understand. Your back leg straight but not locked, your feet correctly positioned and your upper torso in line with your back leg. Repeat the exercise again, with the improved positioning. You should find that your partner can push you much harder before you start to buckle.

The Bow Stance should also be stable from a pull. This time try a similar exercise but with your arm extended. Your partner should gently grab your wrist and pull it.

You will find that if your knee extends too far over your ankle, they can pull you easily. This can be corrected by ensuring that your shinbone is nearly vertical and that your knee is directly above your ankle. This will allow you to resist their pull more easily.

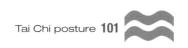

Empty Stance

The Empty Stance is tested in the same way as the Bow Stance.

Foot Position

The position of your feet is just as important in the Empty Stance as it is in the Bow Stance. Try the following to prove it to yourself.

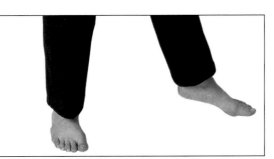

1 In the Empty Stance, your leading foot should be either in line with the back heel or just off to the left (if you are standing on your right leg).

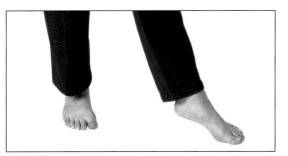

2 Do it deliberately wrong and cross your stance by placing your leading foot to the right of the line of your right heel.

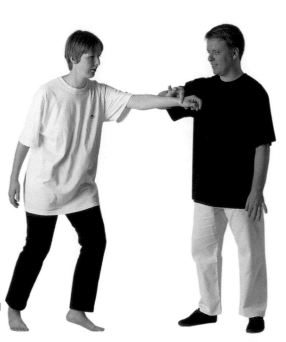

3 Your training partner should then push on your shoulder or pull your arm lightly. You will soon overbalance. The reason for this is that you cannot sink to counteract their force. Try it again in the correct position and feel the difference.

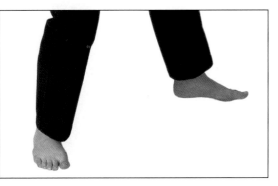

4 The other extreme would be to have your foot too far to the left. Try the exercise again and you will have the same sort of results. Think about how you feel. In the position with your leg so far to the left, it may feel that it is disconnected from the rest of you on some sort of internal level. If you have this feeling, then you are doing well. It means that you are establishing the internal energy connections that will help you with your Tai Chi.

Another exercise concerns the position of your front shin. This exercise will not need repeating many times as it tends to stick quickly.

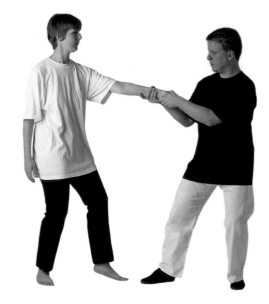

1 Stand in a good Empty Stance. Your partner will pull your arm. You should find it quite easy to ground their efforts through your front leg.

2 Move your front leg back into a position that is closer to your standing leg. This will make the angle of your shin to the floor incorrect. Get your partner to repeat the pull. It will very easy for them to make you overbalance in this position.

Arm and hand positions

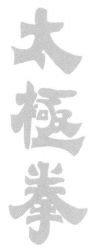

We have so far done a lot of work with the footwork and posture. This is what you would expect when learning Tai Chi, as the hands cannot work properly without getting the feet right.

There are many exercises to help you get the movements perfect. Two of the most popular are the 'unbreakable arm' and the elbow pull. They are designed to prove that there is more to martial arts than brute strength and teach you the correct way of moving your arms.

Unbreakable Arm

This exercise is also popular with other 'soft' styles of martial arts, such as Aikido.

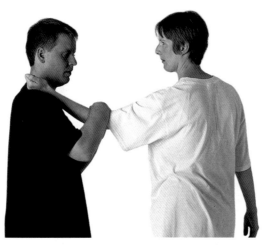 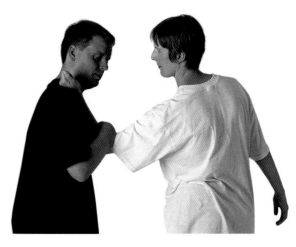

1 Start by standing opposite your training partner and place your hand, palm upwards on their shoulder. Clench your fist as tight as you can and clench your arm muscles.

2 Your partner then tries to push down on your elbow and bend the joint. In this situation, you are using muscular force to stop them. If you are the stronger, you will be able to hold them back for some time. If they are stronger than you, as shown here, it will be impossible to keep your arm straight. When you have experienced the feeling, relax.

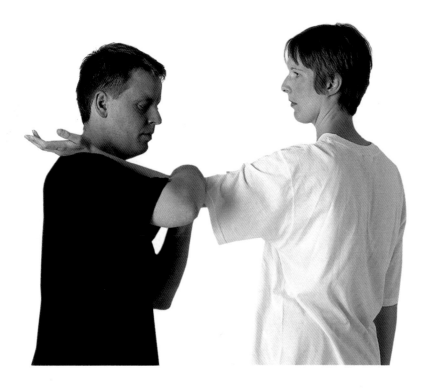

3 Now place your open hand on your partner's shoulder. Keep it relaxed. Imagine that you are extending your intent through your fingertips to a great distance. Keep your muscles relaxed, but your intent strong. Your partner is going to do the same again, but this time you will stop them with your intent. As your partner puts the pressure on, stay relaxed but keep your arm straight with intent. You will find that it is very difficult for them to bend your arm this time.

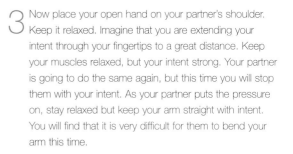

I have shown this exercise to many people. Nobody I have met has been able to give an explanation that does not involve the use of Chi. It seems that this is an exercise that everybody can do that challenges how we understand our bodies.

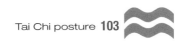

The following exercise works in a similar way.

1 Your partner grabs your extended hand. Try to pull your hand back from their grip. Unless you are stronger, it will be difficult.

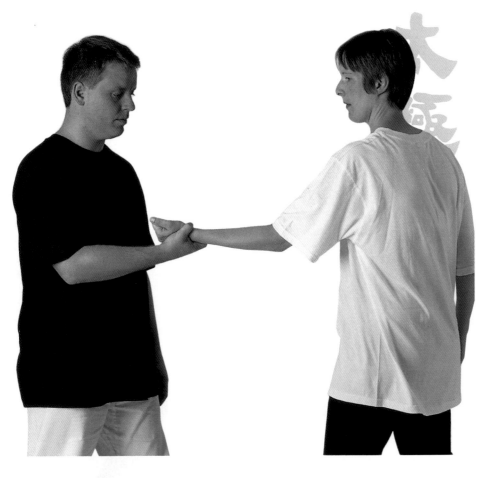

2 Start again with your hand extended, but keep your arm relaxed. Try to forget the fact that somebody has hold of your wrist. Pull back your elbow, not your hand. You will find that it is easy to pull back if you stay relaxed and think about your elbow instead of your hand.

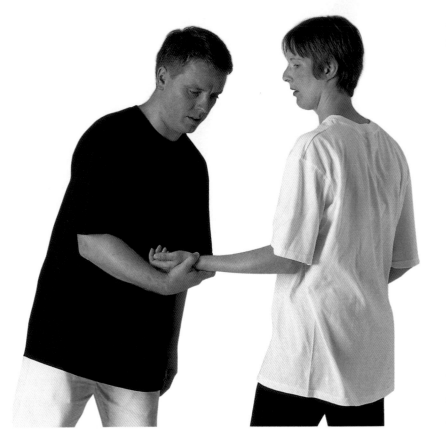

These two quite simple exercises teach you how to work your arms in Tai Chi. Try and think of some more along the same lines. This will help you to improve.

Posture testing

You now have a basic knowledge of how to test your Tai Chi posture. If you can apply this logic to all of your Tai Chi postures you will learn rapidly. This section shows how to apply this knowledge to your Tai Chi form. The following examples are to help you on your way.

1. The Push

Observe all of the points that you have learned from the last exercises. Try the push with both arms extended, one arm extended and your fist clenched. Remember to keep your shoulders and elbows down and gradually build up the strength of the exercise.

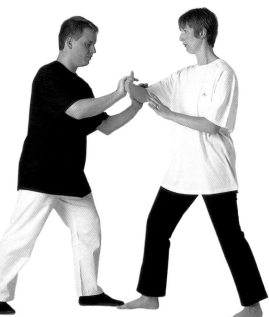

2. Ward-off

This works like the test for the push. Make sure that your training partner pushes against your wrist and elbow.

3. White Crane

A good way to test this posture is to have your partner pull down on your right arm. If you can extend your energy properly you can nearly have them hanging off your arm.

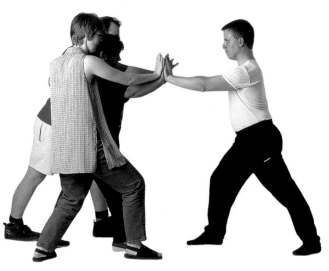

Once you are confident you have mastered correct posture, you could try to practise your skill in a more dramatic way. See how many people you can hold back, simply by using what you have learnt about posture. This is actually a recreation of a famous demonstration by Chen Man Ching.

Posture in motion

When you can understand and do all of these exercises and experiments, it is time to try to put that knowledge into your form. This will take time to integrate so do not rush yourself.

A good indicator of the level of intent is how your hands are used. The following two examples show how the form should be done and how it should not.

In the correct form (figs. 1-4), the fingers are extended but not tight. This allows you to extend your Chi to your fingertips. When your hands come down, your elbows pull back and the energy in your hands stays extended.

In the incorrect form (figs. 5-8), the hands are loose, so the energy cannot fully extend. When lowering, the fingers are limp and the hands come all the way back to the chest.

Right

fig. 1 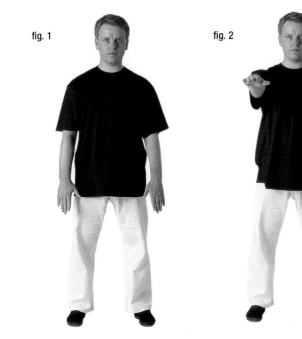 fig. 2 fig. 3 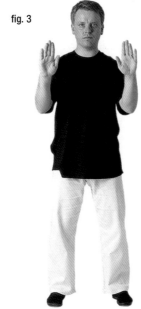 fig. 4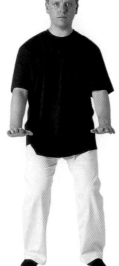

Wrong

fig. 5 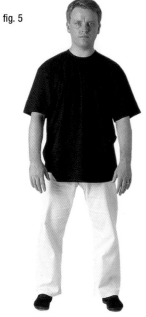 fig. 6 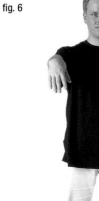 fig. 7 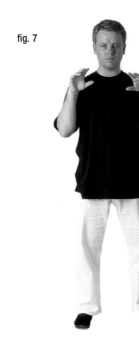 fig. 8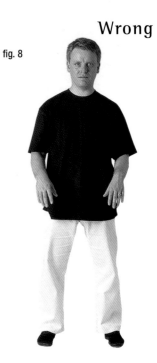

TAI CHI APPLICATIONS

As we have said before, Tai Chi is a martial art. If you are to understand Tai Chi to your full potential you need to understand the martial art side of Tai Chi.

The martial applications of Tai Chi are not theoretical – they do work. The level of their efficacy is determined by the skill of the person doing the move. If executed properly, the Tai Chi techniques are just as effective as the styles that are commonly labelled as 'practical'. Indeed, many styles such as karate and Aikido have utilised some Tai Chi techniques.

A common question that you will see in some magazines is, 'which martial art works best at street level?' Usually Tai Chi will be about last in the list. Those with little or no understanding of the art frequently see it as being slow and ineffective. Do not let these stories distract you. If people ask me the question, I normally reply by saying that I prefer to avoid the possibility of street violence and that I hope to aspire to higher levels than a street fighter!

Another explanation goes back to the first Essence, 'lift the spirit'. Imagine a pack of animals being followed by a hunter. The hunter will pick on the one that is trailing at the back, not the spirited beast that leads the pack. If your spirit is strong, it will show on a subconscious level to a would-be predator and will hopefully deter them.

When practising Tai Chi applications, you need a partner. Remember to tread softly. You do not want to hurt your partner. If your partner has shown enough trust to train with you in this way, you must respect that trust. Do not, however, be too soft. When you practise a technique on someone, they are also learning what it feels like when different people use the technique on them. Neither of you will learn if you do not use the technique properly.

The applications shown here are not definitive. For each movement, there are normally several applications. This is a chance to be creative. If you can think of any more, practise them carefully and see if they work. You will really get to understand your Tai Chi this way because you have started to think for yourself.

Graceful movements, such as White Crane Spreads its Wings, also have many martial applications

Applications for Opening Form

1 Your training partner has grabbed hold of you by the wrists. You can throw them by raising your hands. For this application to work you must stay soft and visualise energy extending past your fingertips.

2 Do not try to use muscular force, which would simply result in the strongest person winning. In Tai Chi applications, assume that your aggressor is stronger than you are. This means that you have to use technique, rather than strength.

3 Your partner may not always be thrown by your raised hands. In this case, you need to lower them again to escape.

4 If your partner keeps hold of you, then they will come crashing into you.

5 To avoid this, torque your waist and they will be thrown past you to the right-hand side.

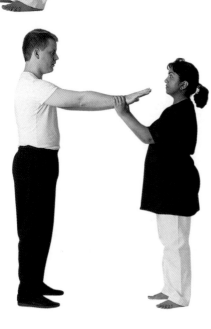
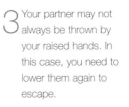
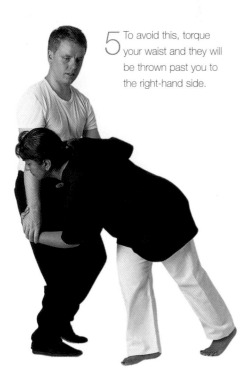

Applications for Grasping the Sparrow's Tail

This sequence contains four different movements and they will be explained individually.

1. Ward-off

1 Your training partner punches towards you with their left fist.

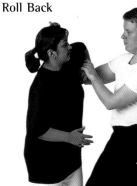

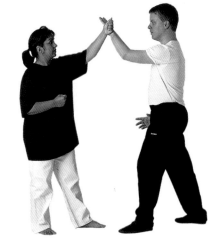

2 Raise the fingers of your left hand to block with your forearm. Do not stop moving once you have started and you will move your forearm around in a circle bringing your partner's fist with it. You will need to keep your arm soft, so that you can stay in contact with your partner.

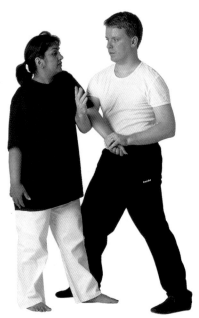

3 When you have brought their fist low, grab it with your left hand to gain control. While you have control of their fist with your left hand, slide your right forearm to meet your partner's elbow in the Ward-off position. When your arms make the Ward-off position, step into the Bow Stance.

You will now have control of your partner's arm by locking the elbow. If you rotate their elbow, it will lift their shoulder and put them off-balance.

Roll Back

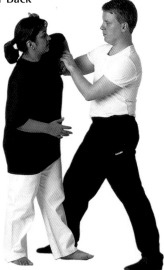

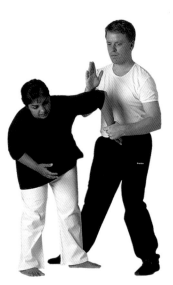

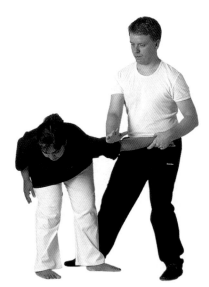

1 The way to escape from the elbow lock in the last move is to lift the elbow before the lock can be executed properly. In Tai Chi we never fight force with more force. Therefore, you will follow the elbow on its journey upwards. If you lift your left hand at the last part of the move, your training patner's shoulder will rise. This will give the control of the situation back to you.

2 If your partner can extend their fingers and push down, they may be able to escape. Again, the solution is not to use force. Just sink your weight back on to your left leg and move into Roll Back. This will cause your partner's arm to be over-extended and locked at the elbow

3 If you were to torque your waist further, you would throw your partner, or break their arm.

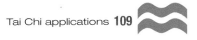

Squeeze

The only option that is open to your training partner now is to try to unlock their elbow and push it into your abdomen. Neutralise this by dropping your right elbow. When you drop your elbow and turn your waist, your left hand comes up to meet your right forearm. This puts you in position for a Squeeze move. Push from your back leg to execute the Squeeze.

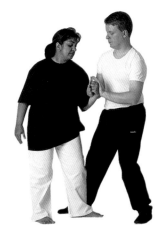

Press

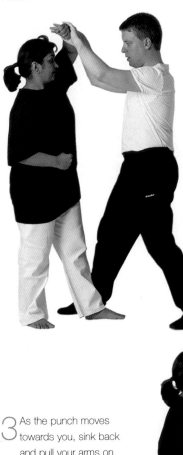

1 Your training partner senses the Squeeze approaching, so they deflect it with an upper block. This forces both of your hands to rise, so they try a punch towards your stomach.

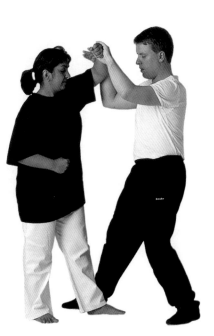

2 When you feel the Squeeze movement rise, separate your hands. This will give you control over their forearm.

3 As the punch moves towards you, sink back and pull your arms on an inward arc. This will use your partner's arm to block his or her own punch.

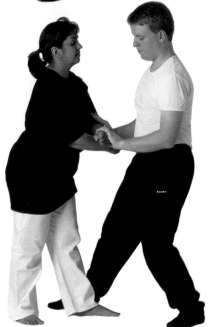

4 From the position where you are set back on your left leg, push forward into the Bow Stance. At the same time extend your arms to push. This double push will push your partner back to complete the sequence.

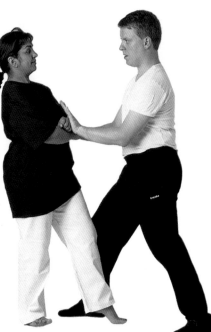

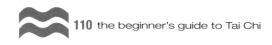

Applications for Single Whip

1 Perhaps your push at the end of the last sequence was neutralised by your training partner's Ward-of movement.

2 You can use the transition movement into Single Whip to throw them.

3 If you connect with your partner's wrist and elbow, you will have the greatest control.

4 Your right hand – the hook – can be used for a strike as shown.

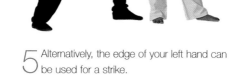

5 Alternatively, the edge of your left hand can be used for a strike.

Application for Raise Hands

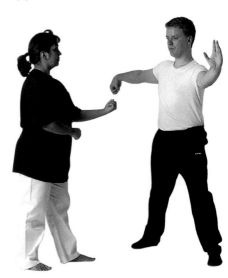

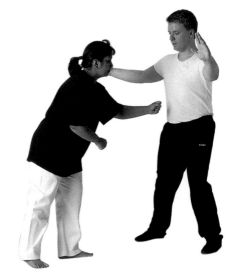

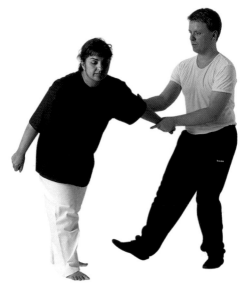

1 From the Single Whip position, your most vulnerable side will be your right. If you can dictate your training partner's attack, you have the advantage of knowing what they are going to do before they do.

2 It is possible to dictate their movement in this way by giving them an attack that is impossible to resist. Opening your arms does this.

3 When they have given you the attack you were waiting for, the Raise Hands posture can be used to block the attack and attack their elbow.

Applications for White Crane

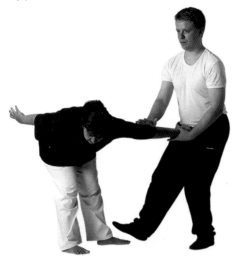 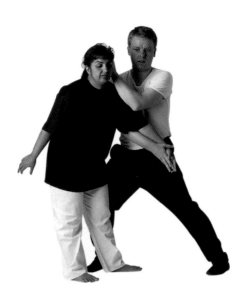 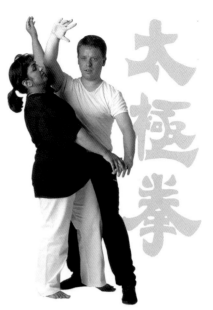 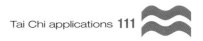

1 If you still have your training partner's wrist and elbow from Raise Hands, you can throw them by sinking.

2 An alternative would be to sink and pull them down so that you can follow through with a strike to their head or neck.

3 After the strike, throw them by stepping up into the White Crane position.

Applications for Brush and Push

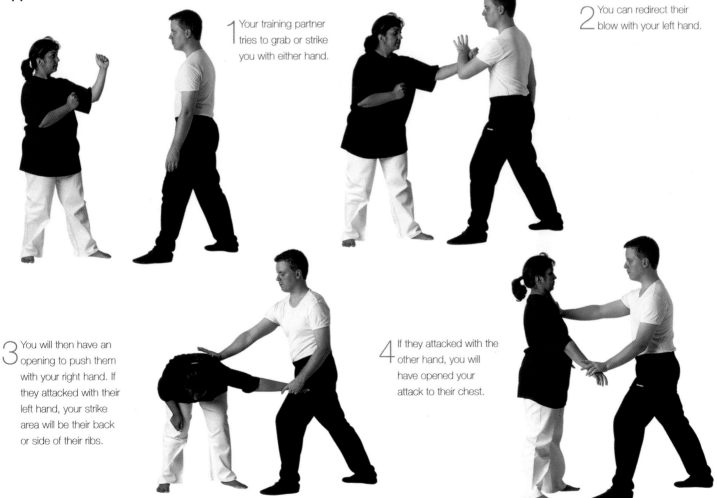

1 Your training partner tries to grab or strike you with either hand.

2 You can redirect their blow with your left hand.

3 You will then have an opening to push them with your right hand. If they attacked with their left hand, your strike area will be their back or side of their ribs.

4 If they attacked with the other hand, you will have opened your attack to their chest.

Application for Strum the Lute

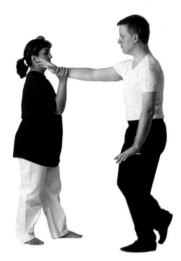 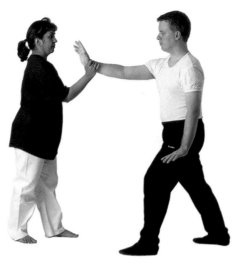 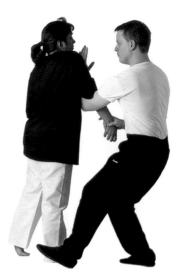

1 Your training partner has hold of your wrist. It could be a continuation from Brush and Push.

2 When they pull against you, do not fight against them. Instead, you should take a half step to them in the direction that they are pulling.

3 This will automatically cause their body to become slacker, and you should then drop your weight into the Empty Stance. As your arms 'Strum the Lute', you will put your partner into an elbow lock.

Applications for Parry, Block and Punch

1 Your training partner punches with their left hand.

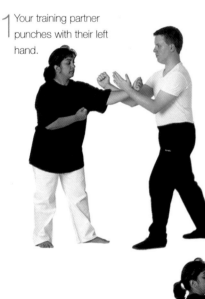

2 You intercept with your left palm and deflect with your right fist.

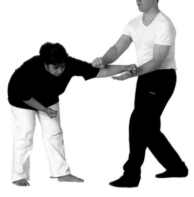

3 Your partner then tries to punch with the right hand.

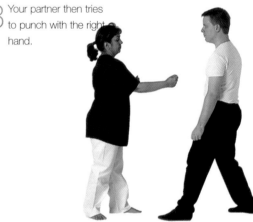

4 Now you block with your left hand. Keep your right fist on the inside of your partner's right fist and they will not be able to strike you.

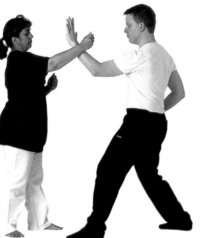

5 Punch to your partner's chest with your right hand. Be sure that the power for the punch is generated from your heel through to your fist.

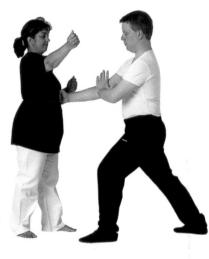

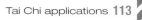

Applications for Apparent Close-up

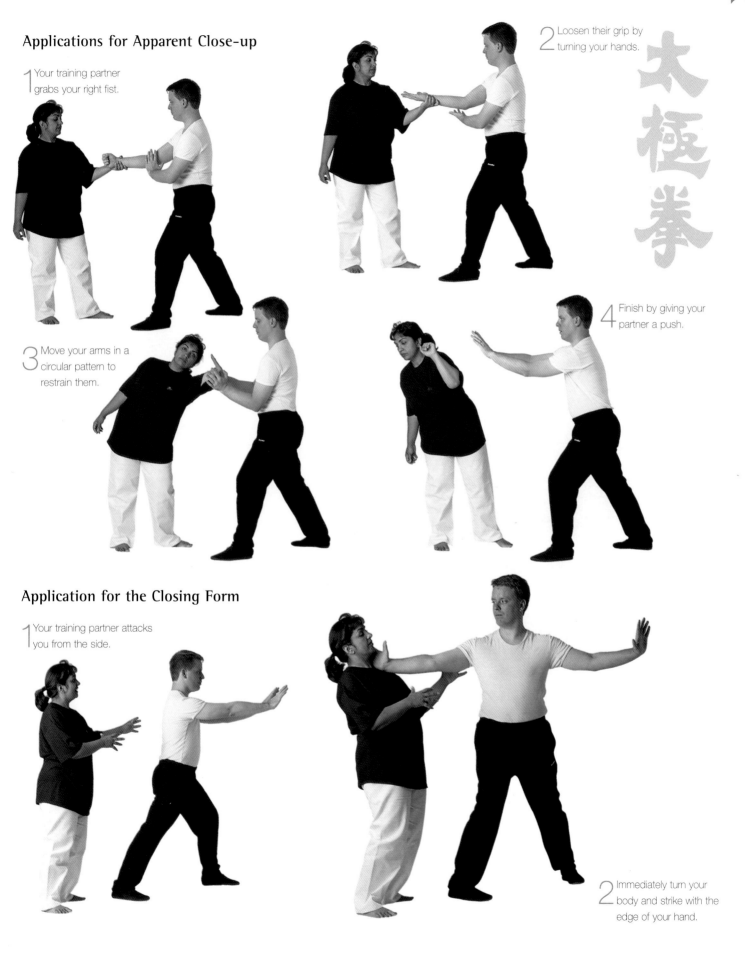

1 Your training partner grabs your right fist.

2 Loosen their grip by turning your hands.

3 Move your arms in a circular pattern to restrain them.

4 Finish by giving your partner a push.

太極拳

Application for the Closing Form

1 Your training partner attacks you from the side.

2 Immediately turn your body and strike with the edge of your hand.

THE TECHNIQUES OR ENERGIES

The full Yang style Tai Chi form is made up of 103 different movements. If they were all completely different it would take many years to learn the sequence alone. Luckily, this is not the case, as within that set of 103 movements, there are only 34 different ones. This is only slightly more comforting as 34 totally different movements will still take a lot of learning.

In those 34 different movements, there are eight different energies or techniques. Of those eight energies, the first four are known as the primary techniques and the second four as the secondary techniques. All of the movements in the form are made from these eight energies or techniques. The eight Energies are:

1. **Ward-off**
2. **Roll Back**
3. **Squeeze**
4. **Press**
5. **Splitting**
6. **Pull Back**
7. **Elbowing**
8. **Leaning**

The first four are the most important in the Yang form, as they appear most frequently. A basic description of each is as follows:

Ward-off

This is the really important one. If you can get your Ward-off movements right, then you are on your way to a good understanding.

Have you seen the trick where somebody gets an egg and squashes it from top to bottom and it does not break? If you have not, then get in the kitchen and try it. The eggshell is very thin but can withstand the pressure because of its physical configuration. This is very similar to the mechanical way that Ward-off works.

Obviously, all of the moves that are called Ward-of, use Ward-off energy. All moves in the form will actually have an element of Ward-off in them.

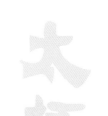

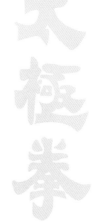

Roll Back

You can get an idea of how Roll Back works if you imagine that the egg from our Ward-off energy had uniform strength all the way round. If you put it under strain, it would exhibit the Ward-off energy. If you were to tilt it slightly, it would spin, and the entire load trying to crush it would be thrown to one side. This is also how a ball bearing works.

Roll Back energy is very similar. It follows Ward-off and then deflects the energy to one side.

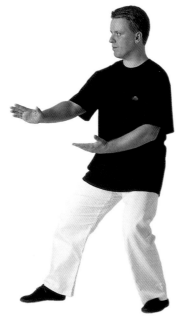

Squeeze

Next time you see a Newton's Cradle toys, take a look at it. It consists of a series of balls suspended on wires. When you pull one back and let go, it strikes the front one and kinetic energy transfers through the lines of balls to the last one, which moves away.

This is the mechanical equivalent of Squeeze energy. Another example could be a stonemason striking his chisel with a mallet so that the energy transfers through the chisel to break the stone.

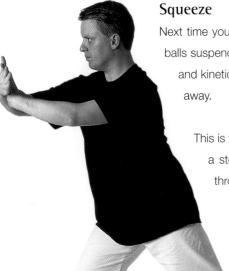

Press

Imagine a spring being compressed and suddenly released. This is how Press works. If your spring were rooted into the floor, all of the energy would be transferred forwards and none wasted. This is also true in Tai Chi. If your feet are rooted into the floor, you will be able to push more energy out with Press.

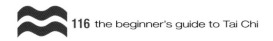

Splitting

This is not used in section one of the form. Its energy is similar to tearing a piece of paper.

Pull Back

This is used in Strum the Lute. Its motion is similar to that of a fishing line being reeled in on a modern reels that uses levers for greater efficiency.

Elbowing

Again, this is not used in section one of the form and is seldom used in the whole of the Yang form. Its effect is quite descriptive – you use your elbow for a strike. It appears more in the Chen style, illustrated here.

Leaning

The only example of leaning in the Yang form is at the transition between Raise Hands and White Crane Spreads its Wings. You use the whole of your body for the movement but do not actually lean over as the name suggests. If an expert does it to you it feels like being hit by a bus.

TWO PERSON PRACTICE DRILLS

When you have learned how to do the form to the level where you no longer have to struggle with the sequence, you are ready to start learning two person practice drills or 'Pushing Hands' as they are commonly known. Pushing Hands will teach you how to use your body properly in the form. You can then feed your improved skill back into your form, which will, in turn, improve your Pushing Hands.

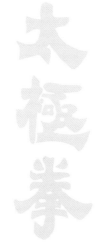

Do not get confused with what we mean here by Pushing Hands. It is a gentle way of practising Tai Chi with a fellow student with no risk of injury to either party. It has a cyclic motion and involves the interplay between your energy and your training partner's energy. It is also non-competitive.

The Pushing Hands that you sometimes see in tournaments is very different to that being explained here. In that event, the competitors will try to push each other over. It frequently involves the use of strength rather than the use of skill.

When practising Pushing Hands, it is possible to be lulled into a relaxed state where your mind switches off. Beware of this, as if it happens you are no longer using intent, so your training is not 100 per cent focused. Always try to get the most out of your Pushing Hands sessions as this is your opportunity to try to get to the core of Tai Chi.

When you execute a push in the Pushing Hands sequences, do not be deceived by its slow speed. As in any Tai Chi movement, you use the whole of your body to put the power into the push.

The slow speed allows you to learn how to open up your body and push the energy forward. Similarly, when yielding, you will use the whole of your body to sink on to your back leg. This body movement is centred at the Tan Tien. When you become accustomed to Pushing Hands practice, you will learn how to perceive the Tan Tien as the centre of movement.

After that, you will actually be able to feel the rota-tions of your Tan Tien. If you can put this feeling into your form without ruining everything else that you have achieved, you will have reached an advanced level.

The beginner will frequently ask, 'Am I doing it right?' A hint here is that if it makes your legs ache, you are on the right track. Practising pushing hands is surprisingly strenuous on the legs. When you think about all of the weight shifting that you are doing it will make more sense. It is always a good idea to stretch after hard work like this. It will help you to stay supple and your legs will ache less in the morning. If you are really suffering, a hot bath is always a good way to finish a hard practice session!

Pushing Hands comes in many different forms. It can be fixed-step, or moving-step when you become advanced. Some of the basic fixed-step pushing hands sequences are explained here.

Pushing Hands theory

In Tai Chi, whether you are practising the form or Pushing Hands, you need to understand the concept of yielding. We have already said that you do not meet force with force, otherwise the strongest would always win. If we do not use strength, then what do we use?

The answer is that we must yield to the oncoming force. Pushing Hands is the ideal place to learn the concept of yielding. Try the following exercises.

Using strength

1 Stand opposite your training partner. Your partner is ready to push you.

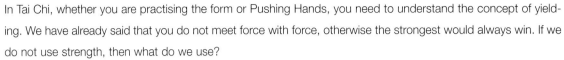

2 As your partner pushes you, fight back by rooting into the floor. Hold your position solid and do not let your partner push you.

As you can see, this creates a situation where the strongest will win. You are both locked on the spot and you are going nowhere. This is not what you would do in Tai Chi. Now try the next exercise.

Using yielding

This is the basic concept of yielding. Note how it requires less effort than trying to use force and it allows you to take control of your partner.

The first Pushing Hands exercise uses the same movement. In the part at the end of the push where you could have thrown your partner you should change from yielding to pushing. Remember Yin and Yang.

When you change from Yin to Yang, it gives you the chance to practise both energies in a cyclic way. Remember that all your power should be rooted from the heel and gradually applied. Pushing Hands can be great fun and very informative.

Which did you find the easiest, Yin or Yang? Is there an imbalance between Yin and Yang in your form? Is giving easier than receiving? Are Yin and Yang balanced in your life? Many questions can be inspired by Pushing Hands practice.

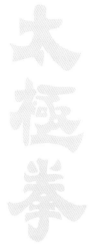

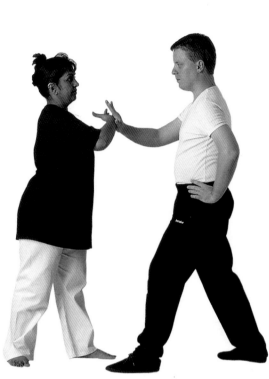

1 Start in a similar position as for the first exercise. Your training partner is ready to push you.

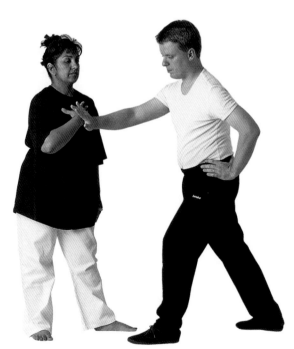

2 As you feel the push, do not fight it, let it come in to you. Yield to the push. Let the push come all the way. It does not matter if your inner forearm touches your own body.

3 When you have let the push come in as far as possible, turn your body. This will redirect your partner's force and you could then throw them if you wanted.

Single-Handed Pushing Hands

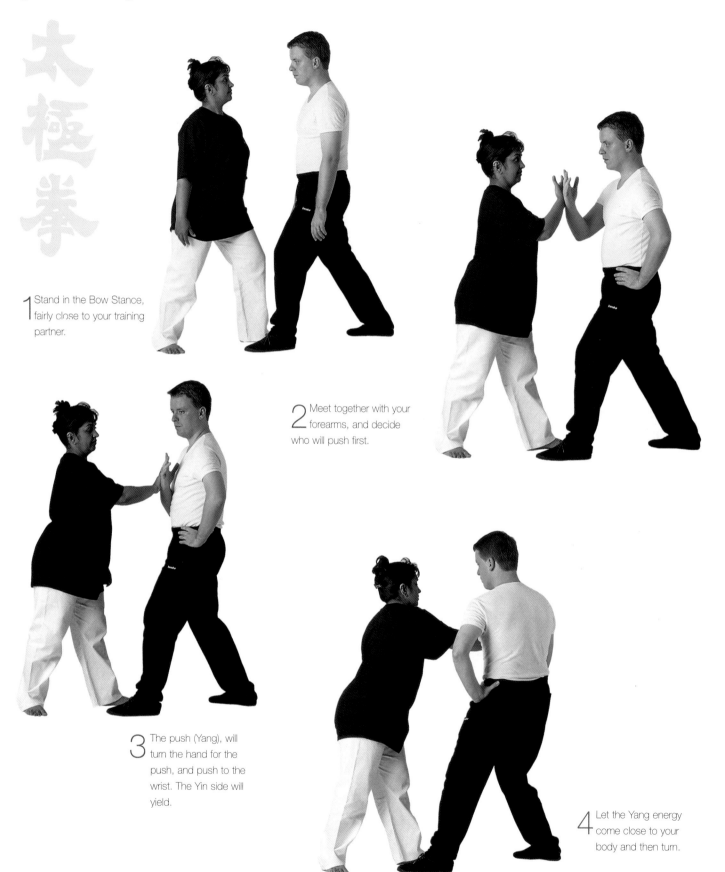

1 Stand in the Bow Stance, fairly close to your training partner.

2 Meet together with your forearms, and decide who will push first.

3 The push (Yang), will turn the hand for the push, and push to the wrist. The Yin side will yield.

4 Let the Yang energy come close to your body and then turn.

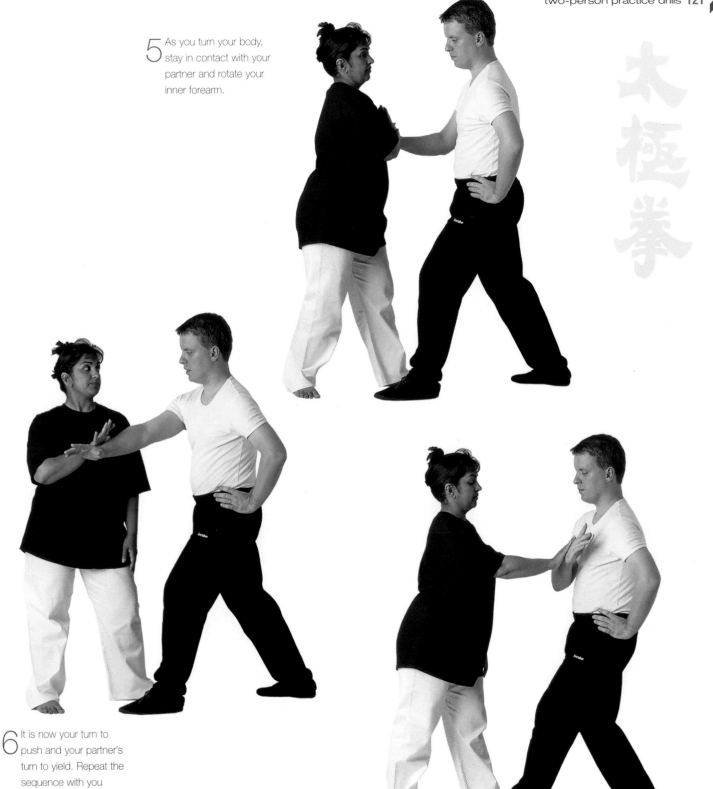

5 As you turn your body, stay in contact with your partner and rotate your inner forearm.

6 It is now your turn to push and your partner's turn to yield. Repeat the sequence with you pushing and your partner yielding.

7 Keep the movement going. You are now practising pushing hands.

Remember that you must stay relaxed. Keep the speed steady and even. Keep your shoulders down. Use weight transfer from one leg to the other to power the movement.

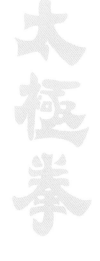

Two-Handed Push

When you can do the single-handed push, it is easy to expand the idea to a two-handed push. Try the following exercise to help you understand how it works.

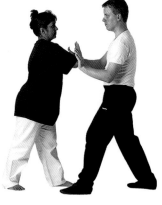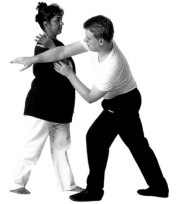

1 Position your training partner so that they are ready to practise the two-hand push. Meet the push with your Ward-off arm.

2 When the push starts to come in, drop your elbow. This will ruin the alignment of your partner's push.

3 You can then yield and push your partner to one side.

The easiest way to start this Pushing Hands routine is to attach it to your single-handed push routine as follows:

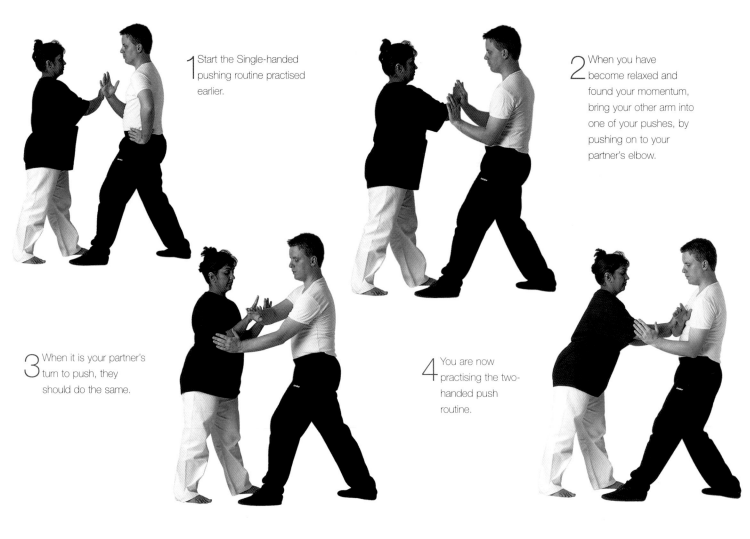

1 Start the Single-handed pushing routine practised earlier.

2 When you have become relaxed and found your momentum, bring your other arm into one of your pushes, by pushing on to your partner's elbow.

3 When it is your partner's turn to push, they should do the same.

4 You are now practising the two-handed push routine.

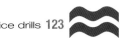

Brush and Push

With imagination, it is possible to transform many of the Tai Chi movements into Pushing Hands routines. This will help you to understand what it is like to apply the movements to a situation where you are training with a partner. Without this, the routine can lack depth.

One of the more straightforward parts of the routine to give this sort of attention to is the Brush and Push sequence, as follows:

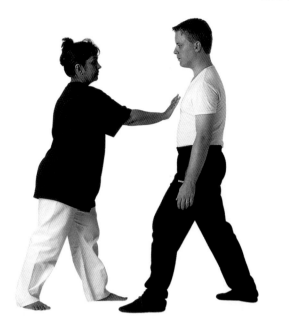

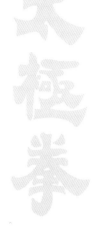

1 Your training partner pushes to you with the right hand.

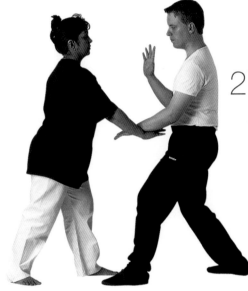

2 You will deflect with your inner left forearm. Simultaneously, you prepare your right hand for the push.

3 Deflect your partner's push with your left arm and push with your right.

4 Your partner will then deflect and push in exactly the same way you just did.

5 Repeat the actions for the routine.

When you have mastered pushing with one arm, you should practise with the other before moving on to the next exercise. Remember that learning Pushing Hands is a slow process and that there are many subtleties that you will only find after repeated practise.

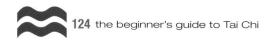

ADVICE ON PRACTICE

Masters such as Yang Chengfu and his sons have had the advantage of being immersed in a martial arts culture with excellent teachers and time to practise their forms. You really would be reaching for the stars if you were to want to compare yourself to them. In our modern world, we sometimes find it difficult to make time for the things that we really want to do. This means that you have to get the most out of the time that you do have. The only way to do this is by ensuring that you practise correctly.

The best way to learn is to get into a class with a good teacher. Train at least a little bit every day. If you do not, then you will keep going over the same old things and you will become bored. Keep yourself and your teacher interested by adding a little bit every day if you can. Even if you cannot physically practise the form, you could go through it in your mind or practise some meditation.

Do not try to do it all at once. Learn how to get through the form. When you can get through the form without memory problems, concentrate on one movement for as long as you can. With repetition, you will find depth in the activity that you can then apply to other movements.

Use what you have got. You may not have the cultural background in martial arts that some of the masters have had, but they never had as much access to information as you. Read magazines, other books, look at videos, visit web sites and visit other clubs. If your intent is genuine, then you will not go far wrong. If you can do everything in this book reasonably well, then you no longer need classify yourself as a complete beginner. Never let the idea of being a beginner totally escape you. A beginner is like an empty cup and it is easier for a master to fill it with knowledge than a full one.

When you can complete section one of the form to a good level, you will be ready to move on to section two. This is normally taught in two parts. It contains many new movements, but they are all based upon the core ideas that you have learned in section one. So you can see that without a good understanding of section one, there is little point in trying section two.

Along with section two, you will need to understand more about the martial side of Tai Chi. Pushing Hands and application practice will help you here.

When you are ready for section three, you will already know most of the movements. You will continue developing your martial arts skills, but you will also need to work on the spiritual side of Tai Chi as well. Meditation practice is useful at this stage, so it is good to have started meditation when you were learning section one.

After you have finished with hand forms, you may choose to learn how to use weapons such as the sword and sabre. Weapons training will teach you a new level of accuracy and intent.

The most important things to remember are:

1. Keep at it – don't give up.
2. Enjoy it!

If you enjoy your Tai Chi as much as I have done over the years, then you will be on to something good.

Snake Creeps Down from Section 3.

Kick with Right Heel from Section 2 and 3.

Punch to Seven Stars from section 3.

INDEX

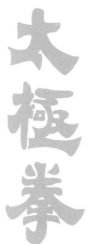

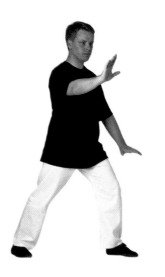

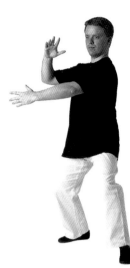

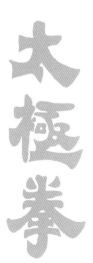

CREDITS AND ACKNOWLEDGEMENTS

I would like to thank my teachers Shelagh Grandpierre and Christopher Pei of the Tai Chi Alliance and the United States Wushu Academy for teaching me what I know about Yang style and Chun Chen of the Universe Tai Chi Society for starting me off and also for some of the warm-up exercises.

Last and most important, I would like to thank my wife Carol for her love and support.

The author and publisher would also like to thank the models that took part in this book: Lisa, Sarah and Colin.

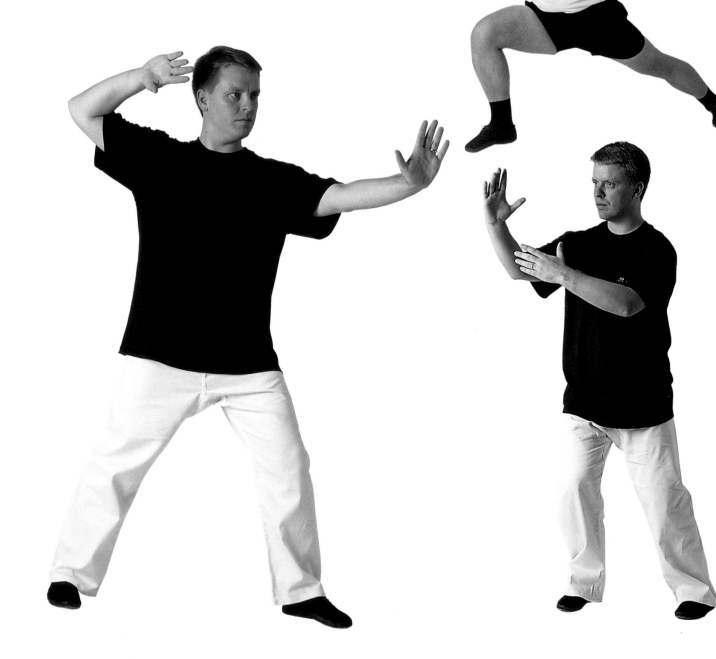